Optimizing Clinical Team Productivity and Quality

2nd Edition

Sheila Richmeier, MS, RN, FACMPE

Medical Group Management Association
104 Inverness Terrace East
Englewood, CO 80112-5306
877.275.6462
mgma.org

MGMA

Medical Group Management Association ®

Library of Congress Cataloging-in-Publication Data
Names: Richmeier, Sheila, author.
MGMA (Association); publisher.
EGZ Publications; production.
Title: Optimizing clinical team productivity and quality / Sheila Richmeier.
Other titles: Leading your clinical team
Description: 2nd. Englewood, CO : Medical Group Management Association,
 [2016] Preceded by: Leading your clinical team / Sheila Richmeier.
 c2010. Includes bibliographical references and index.

Identifiers:
LCCN 2016032708 (print)
LCCN 2016033599 (ebook)

MGMA product id 9027/e9027

PRINT ISBN 978-1-56829-475-9
DIGITAL ISBN 978-1-56829-480-3

Subjects: | MESH: Nursing, Team–organization & administration | Efficiency,
 Organizational | Quality Assurance, Health Care–organization &
 administration
Classification: LCC R728 (print) | LCC R728 (ebook) | NLM WY 125 | DDC
 610.68–dc23

Printed in the United States of America
10 9 8 7 6 5 4 3 2 1

Contents

Chapter 1

Introduction

Most practice administrators are hired because of their proficiency in financial and business office matters. Successful administrators have a solid foundation in accounting, finance, and general business. They also have the expertise to manage revenue and expenses to maximize profit; they understand the nuances of third-party reimbursement, insurance processing, and governmental regulations; they have a background in human resource management as well as leadership principles; and they may be very astute at managing operations.

Ironically, the practice of medicine is all about the clinical side, and effective management of the clinical aspects of medical practice, while imperative, is rarely explored. In today's world, reimbursement for medicine is changing to a more quality- and value-based focus. And it's important, now more than ever, to use all staff effectively, both clinical and non-clinical. This requires a more in-depth knowledge of the clinical side for both business managers and clinical managers.

WHY THIS BOOK?

After physician and administrator salaries, nursing salaries are the highest expense in a practice. This book addresses the implications of poorly coordinating nursing staff activities, and shares suggestions for implementing efficient and effective clinical operations, allowing the practice to focus on quality.

Inefficiency and inadequate resource management cost the practice money. Some nonclinical managers choose to direct their practice with a hands-off approach—assuming whatever nursing asks for, it must need. Some managers try to handle clinical staff as they do office staff. Neither approach is optimal; clinical management is different from nonclinical office/practice management. This book was written to assist nonclinical managers as well as clinical managers in effectively directing the clinical side of the practice. Who are the "right staff" for the clinical aspects of the practice? What measures can be employed to ensure a clinical department operates efficiently? How does the practice administrator know what is "right" or "wrong" without a clinical background? This book provides guidance on these and many other issues.

WHO WILL BENEFIT?

All managers—new or experienced, with or without a clinical background—will find the information in this book to be a quick overview as well as a resource providing many suggestions to measure and improve office efficiency. This book also can be used as a reference for when clinical issues arise. Seasoned clinical managers will find in this volume suggestions to improve their management of the clinical area and will gain knowledge   on nursing staff options and productivity measures, and assistance in developing key clinical supervision know-how.

WHAT IS INCLUDED?

Clinical management of a medical practice starts with understanding personnel and what nursing actually does in a practice. This basic foundation provides insight as production, efficiency, and supervision of nursing are explored. Additional clinical resources, documentation, regulation components, and ancillary services are considered as they affect overall management. This updated version will assist the practice in being successful in an ever-changing world.

The chapters are outlined as follows:

Chapter 2: The Right Staff. Nursing is defined by education and licensure. Differentiating between licensed and non-licensed staff, experience, and pay differences are explored.

Chapter 3: Nursing Functions in a Medical Practice. This chapter defines nursing functions provided in a medical office, identifies the differences among specialties, and makes suggestions for the use of licensed vs. non-licensed staff. Beginning discussions of the team are initiated.

Chapter 4: Staff Accountability. Productivity and outcomes are used to assist in determining staffing, and examples are given. Although using one measure provides some data in determining productivity, using several different measures creates a more comprehensive assessment.

Chapter 5: Clinical Efficiency. Pre-visit, visit, and post-visit activities are analyzed in depth to explore opportunities for improvement. Suggestions to maximize efficiency are shared.

Chapter 6: Supervision of Nursing Staff. Who supervises clinical staff in a medical practice, the administrator or the physician? The process of delegating nursing responsibilities and determining who ultimately supervises clinical staff is clarified. Training and competency are defined in developing the nursing role.

Chapter 7: The Right Amount of Staff. Following the discussion of how to utilize the productivity measures in Chapter 4, this chapter expands on using those measures to assess staffing levels. Benchmarking is explained, including a specific clinic example, and different nursing models are defined.

Chapter 8: Clinical Supply Resources. Management of clinical supplies in a medical practice requires some attention. This chapter identifies tips for managing pharmaceutical and medical supplies, equipment, forms, and patient education materials.

Chapter 9: Documentation. Documentation is a very important component of nursing practice. Most nurses learn documentation in a hospital setting, and the differences between that and medical practice nursing are explored.

Chapter 10: Regulations. Regulations such as those mandated by the Occupational Safety and Health Administration, the Health Insurance Portability and Accountability Act, and the Centers for Disease Control and Prevention affect nursing care in a medical practice. An overview of regulations is provided along with suggestions for implementation. Clinical research is also explained in relation to regulatory issues.

Chapter 11: Other Management Issues. This chapter explores the role of the nurse in the hospital setting as it differs from that in the medical practice. The change in mentality from hospital to medical office is significant. The nurse-physician relationship is explored, and other management issues are discussed.

Chapter 12: Ancillary Services. Other departments in the medical practice include diagnostic testing, modalities other than nursing, and retail. This chapter briefly touches on how the other parts of the book can be used to identify staffing needs, implement efficiency measures, tighten documentation processes, and meet regulations in the ancillary departments.

Chapter 13: Advanced Practice. Midlevel providers are sometimes caught between staff and physicians. This chapter defines their education, their role, and the costs and benefits they represent to the practice.

FINAL THOUGHTS

This book is relevant for any size practice because all practices have a clinical side. There are numerous right ways to manage the clinical side and many aspects are included within this book... Both clinical and nonclinical managers may find this book very useful in making their practice more efficient or cost effective. The clinical staff provide a huge benefit to any practice, and managing them effectively reaps many rewards.

Chapter 2

The Right Staff

Have you ever looked at the spectrum of clinical staff—licensed or non-licensed, experienced or inexperienced, certified or noncertified, registered or practical—and wondered how it all fits together? The myriad options available for nursing professionals to pursue are confusing even for those managers with clinical experience.

Achieving the "right" clinical staff in a medical practice or clinic depends on many factors, including the type, size, and needs of the practice. The type of medical specialty often dictates clinical staffing. For instance, a primary care clinic will not require a surgical technologist, an ophthalmology practice will probably not need to staff a registered nurse (RN), and so forth. The size of the practice will also have an impact on staffing needs. Understanding what the clinical staff can contribute to the practice and what needs exist in the practice itself will help better identify staffing requirements.

TYPES OF NURSING STAFF

Physician practices essentially employ two types of clinical staff: licensed and non-licensed.

LICENSED STAFF

Licensed nursing staff are regulated by a state agency, often called the board of nursing. This licensing body defines nursing practice by way of its nurse practice act, which establishes how the nursing board regulates the practice of nursing and nursing education. Most importantly, the board of nursing defines the term nursing itself. For example, one state's Nurse Practice Act defines nursing in the following way:

The practice of professional nursing as performed by a registered professional nurse for compensation or gratuitously… means the process in which substantial specialized knowledge derived from the biological, physical, and behavioral sciences is applied to: the care, diagnosis, treatment, counsel and health teaching of persons who are experiencing changes in the normal health processes or who require assistance in the maintenance of health or the prevention or management of illness, injury or infirmity; administration, supervision or teaching of the process as defined in this section; and the execution of the medical regimen as prescribed by a person licensed to practice medicine and surgery or a person licensed to practice dentistry.[1]

In addition to establishing its definition for nursing, many Nurse Practice Acts define licensed practical nurse (LPN). It is important for clinic managers to know and understand the regulations as they relate to the practice of nursing in their state. These can be obtained by typing "board of nursing" into any Internet search engine and locating the state website in which the practice is located. For those organizations requiring a nurse to practice in two states simultaneously , both states' regulations should be reviewed. Although all states regulate nursing in their unique way, similarities among them exist. Most state practice acts include requirements for the following:

- Protection of the public
- Licensure requirements for competence in nursing practice
- Accountability for conduct
- Educational requirements of nursing schools

Protection of the Public

The title of nurse is limited to those practitioners who comply with the state regulations for the protection of the public. Identifying yourself as a nurse is illegal if you are not licensed as a nurse. False identification misrepresents the caregiver's educational background and experience to patients. They may think they are dealing with a nurse when in actuality they may be interacting with a medical assistant. Nursing and office staff must be careful to clarify this differentiation with the public.

---

1 Kansas State Board of Nursing. Kansas Nurse Practice Act. www.ksbn.org. (Accessed 10/3/08 and 2.28.2016)

The following example demonstrates the improper use of the term nurse: In a general surgery practice, a patient was told by the telephone attendant that she needed to speak with a nurse but was transferred to a surgical technologist. The patient mistakenly assumed she was talking with a nurse. Although the surgical technologist was very good at his job, the practice essentially lied to this patient and led her to believe she was talking to someone with the knowledge, education, and experience of a nurse.

Licensure Requirements

Registered nurses or practical nurses are considered licensed staff and are licensed through the state's board of nursing. The state's nurse practice act defines licensure requirements, including fees, qualifications, successfully completed examinations and refresher courses, and titles.

In general, nursing offers several entry levels to practice, from a one-year technical degree to a four-year bachelor's degree and beyond. Nursing staff are identified by the initials (degree abbreviations) that follow their name. Degrees in the field of nursing, and their abbreviations, include those listed in **Exhibit 2.1**.

EXHIBIT 2.1	Nursing Degrees and Their Abbreviations		
RN	Registered nurse	PhD	Doctor of philosophy, nursing major
LPN	Licensed practical nurse	DNP	Doctor of nursing practice
LVN	Licensed vocational nurse	FNP	Family nurse practitioner
BSN	Bachelor's degree in nursing	ARNP	Advanced registered nurse practitioner
MS	Master of science, nursing major	NP	Nurse practitioner
MSN	Master of science in nursing	CNS	Clinical nurse specialist
ADN	Associate's degree in nursing	CRNA	Certified registered nurse anesthetist

Licensure for each entry level is as follows:

- Licensed practical nurse (LPN)/licensed vocational nurse (LVN). The education required to achieve LPN/LVN status is usually a one- or two-year program that prepares the individual to sit for the practical nurse licensure exam after completion. Licensed practical nurses are trained in the technical side of nursing: administering medications, performing treatments, and assisting in the care of the patient. They are supervised by an RN. Licensed practical nurses usually do not practice independently without a supervising RN.

- Associate degree registered nurse (ADN). Registered nurses completing this two-year program are awarded a degree and the ability to take the RN licensure exam. The graduate is qualified to provide and manage patient care in the hospital, home, or clinic setting upon completion.

- Diploma-prepared registered nurse. Although this approach was a very popular way to train RNs many years ago, only one or two programs are still available in the United States. The individual trained in such a program is employed by the hospital as the hospital prepares him or her to become a nurse. The focus of this training is patient care. The successful candidate is awarded a diploma upon completion, which allows him or her to take the registered nurse licensure exam.

- Bachelor's degree RN with a major in nursing (BSN). This RN has been trained in nursing but also has a more well-rounded general education. Emphasis is placed on critical thinking, theory, and management of patients and other staff. The graduate is eligible to take the registered nurse licensure exam.

- Master's degree/doctoral degree. Advanced education in nursing is available in fields such as education, administration, and clinical applications. Advanced registered nurses are all trained for independent and collaborative practice. RN licensure is usually obtained prior to entering these degree programs.

- Chapter 13 more fully explores the role of the advanced practice nurse.

- A comparison of nursing roles (**Exhibit 2.2**) shows the differences in education, licensure, and preparation for each.

After an individual has completed a course of education for either the RN or LPN/LVN program, he or she must write to the board of nursing and request permission to take the board examination (boards). Each state regulates nursing education and requirements to take the boards, and it regulates the retaking of the exam if an individual does not pass on first or subsequent attempts. Nurses who are waiting to take boards may work as a graduate practice nurse (for LPN) or a graduate nurse (for RN). If supervised, they may perform all the functions of an LPN or RN, respectively. When they pass boards, they are then called LPN/ LVN or RN. If they fail boards, they can no longer work in the capacity of a nurse and can be employed only as a nursing assistant until they pass the exam. Each state regulates how many times an individual may take the boards before being required to take additional training or to reapply.

EXHIBIT 2.2	Comparison of Nursing Roles		
Role	Educational Requirements	Abilities	Other
LPN/LVN	1 to 2- year vocational degree	Care for patient - technical component Administer medications, perform treatments, assist in care of patient	Requires supervision by RN
RN - ADN	2-year associate's degree	Provide and manage patient care, including IV therapy	
RN - diploma	3-year diploma	Provide and manage patient care, including IV therapy	Education provided by hospital program
RN - BSN	4-year bachelor's degree	Critical thinking, theory and management of patients and staff	
RN-MS or MSN	6-year master's degree	Advanced degree may be in administration, nurse practitioner, nurse anesthetist, nurse clinician, nurse midwife, health care informatics, organizational leadership, public health nursing, or other	
RN - doctorate	8 to 10- year doctoral degree	DNP - doctor of nursing practice in advanced practice or leadership PhD - doctor of philosophy in nursing	DNP new for nursing

Nurses have to be licensed in the state in which they will practice and can hold licenses from more than one state simultaneously as long as they meet the licensure requirements from each state. A temporary license is issued while the state verifies the licensure of that individual.

Licensure requires a fee be paid every one to two years to the state board of nursing. Some states require continuing education hours to maintain licensure, while others do not. Whether continuing education is required is stated in the nurse practice act of each state.

Accountability for Conduct

The nurse practice act defines standards of practice for nursing, unlawful acts, and unprofessional conduct. These definitions usually include the handling of complaints, disciplinary procedures, and licensure restrictions.

Licensure verification can be done through most boards of nursing for a fee. If you are not able to verify a potential nursing staff member's licensure using past employment records, licensure verification with the state is a good alternative. Each month, nursing boards also report any disciplinary actions and/or suspensions of nursing licenses on their website or through a monthly publication.

Because the nursing boards for each state regulate the practice of nursing, any employer of a nurse found to be acting in a manner that falls outside the nurse practice act must report that incident to the board of nursing for the state where the act occurred. Examples of such breaches are a nurse self-prescribing narcotic medication, helping himself or herself to narcotics, or willfully harming a patient. Once an incident is reported, the board sets up a hearing at which the nurse is given parameters of conduct to follow to remain licensed. Failure to adhere to these parameters results in the loss of the license.

Licensure is a very serious matter, and rightfully so. It should never be taken lightly because obtaining a nursing license requires considerable work.

Educational Requirements of Nursing Schools

Nurse practice acts define the approval process for nursing schools, including the requirements of the curriculum, facilities, and faculty. Surveys are conducted by the state to ensure requirements have been met.

NON-LICENSED CLINICAL STAFF

States differ in how they regulate the practice of nursing and roles related to nursing. Often times they need to clarify the role of the non-licensed clinical staff and publish position statements thatfurther define nursing. They usually are developed around controversial or hot topic issues such as delegation of duties to non-licensed nursing personnel. This topic is explored in Chapter 6.

Non-licensed staff is an all-encompassing title for anyone providing patient care who neither has, nor requires, a license. This is a broad category with many different titles. In the nursing industry, non-licensed staff are grouped together under the name unlicensed assistive personnel (UAP). These positions range from someone who works in a practice who has completed no formal education program to someone who has completed a specific training related to their role and gained certification. (Note that certification is not the same as licensure.) Some of the most general UAP titles are listed in **Exhibit 2.3.**

EXHIBIT 2.3	Unlicensed Assistive Personnel Titles		
MA	Medical assistant	ORT	Operating room technician
NA	Nursing assistant	HCA	Health care associate
CMA	Certified medical assistant	CP	Care partner
CNA	Certified nursing assistant	ST	Surgical technologist
PCT	Patient care technician	COA	Certified ophthalmic assistant
PCA	Patient care assistant	COT	Certified ophthalmic technician
HHA	Home health aide	COMT	Certified ophthalmic medical technologist

Frequently seen in medical offices are the medical assistant (MA), nursing assistant (NA), or home health aide (HHA). Generally, NAs have completed an 8- to 12-week course that allows them to take a nursing assistant exam. They become a certified nursing assistant upon passing the exam. Nursing assistants should be able to show their diploma to verify their training. Nursing assistant training covers basics of patient care, including how to give a bath, position a patient, assist a patient to move, and take vital signs. Be aware, however, that many people call themselves nursing assistants without having completed training.

The medical assistant program is a more formal course of training, which may be a 10-12 week course or a one- to two-year program. Often it is much more extensive than a nursing assistant course and usually includes technical components such as giving shots and drawing blood. Medical assistants are typically trained in office functions such as medical record-keeping and front desk duties. They will have either an associate's degree or a diploma from a medical assistant school. Some become certified after training.

Home health aides are usually certified nursing assistants who have additional training as defined by each state. The focus, of course, is on taking care of the patient in the home setting. Once again, an HHA should have a certificate of completion from an appropriate program.

Each specialty has different certification, identified by designated letters following the person's name. Various certification programs exist for different specialties. General surgery, for instance, includes surgical technologists who complete a one- to two-year course on surgery.

The Centers for Medicare and Medicaid Services (CMS) has tried to clarify roles by stating that "clinical staff" need to be credentialed outside of the practice setting to enter medication, laboratory and radiology orders into the computerized provider order entry (CPOE) system for meaningful use. Make sure and check these regulations prior to assigning responsibilities.[2]

The many types of unlicensed assistive personnel can create confusion, as when a potential employee applies for a position claiming certification in a specialty whose credential initials you do not recognize. Be sure to research the credentials that an applicant lists to determine what their education and certification mean. Ask for a certificate or diploma when the applicant includes such initials following their name. Incongruence may exist between the title claimed and the actual training received. Asking questions and researching credentials are often required. Never hire someone without a full understanding of his or her training and competencies.

2   Stage 2 Eligible Professional Meaningful Use Core Measures Measure 1 of 17 Date issued: October, 2012; https://www.cms.gov/Regulations-and-Guidance/Legislation/EHRIncentivePro-grams/downloads/Stage2_EPCore_1_CPOE_MedicationOrders.pdf; accessed 5.31.2016

EXPERIENCE OF THE NURSING STAFF

Experience is a key factor in determining whether staff will be able to perform their job tasks. It would be difficult for a new graduate nurse to provide telephone triage in a family practice without experience in a hospital setting. Simple nursing situations arise everyday on a medical or surgical hospital floor and this allows the nurse to improve their clinical decision making skills to assist patients. Situations may include simple pain control techniques, managing functional problems with activities of daily living (ADLs), or how to instruct patients on managing their chronic disease more effectively. Many life and practice experiences may also prepare the nurse to handle situations more readily.

Experience can have many benefits for unlicensed staff as well. If a physician has invested time in educating a medical assistant over the course of several years, that MA will know which questions he or she can field and which require the physician's attention. An experienced surgical technologist will be able to answer certain questions more appropriately regarding pain after surgery if he or she has assisted with positioning the patient during surgery and understands the surgical procedure. Often, when they first start in the practice, the new surgical technologists are unable to provide pain-related information to patients because they lack adequate training that comes from experience.

Physician and practice liability are greatly reduced by an experienced nursing staff, especially related to phone triage. A less experienced nurse may give advice to the patient that is detrimental to his or her well-being and results in legal action. The following example demonstrates this issue: In a primary care setting, a nurse has to recognize the signs and symptoms of a heart attack. Patients often experience symptoms other than chest pain, such as indigestion, pain in the shoulder or arm, or shortness of breath that can be indicative of an acute event. If the nurse is not experienced in listening for clues, he or she may not recognize the potentially life-threatening situation. An experienced nurse will initiate emergency procedures when a less experienced nurse may not.

TEAM-BASED CARE

Teams depend on complementary roles to function. For instance, a baseball team requires a pitcher, catcher, outfielders, and basemen. We would not expect the catcher to do the pitching, nor would we expect a baseman to catch pitches. Each player on the team has a specific role to play and it is clearly defined. Teams in medical offices require the same definition and clarity.

The first step in developing an effective team is to define all complementary roles, their scope and functionality. Licensure and experience are key factors in determining the scope and capability of team members. Each team member is responsible to work at the top of their capabilities and to help the team define their role. An example:

A registered nurse (RN) in a medical office has always roomed patients for a physician, but there is a new position needed for care management of high-risk chronic disease patients. As the team starts to determine team roles, the role of the staff member who rooms patients is examined. It is determined that this position does not require the skills and licensure of the RN, but can be carried out by a trained unlicensed clinical staff member. On the other hand, the care management role will require clinical decision making skills and therefore will need to be performed by the RN. The RN is better suited to use her education, experience, and licensure to assist patients with care management of their diseases.

PAY DIFFERENCES

Regardless of the level of experience, education, licensure status, or other factors discussed above, choosing a person to fill a clinical position in a medical practice may come down to how much the practice can afford to pay. Registered nurse compensation is not low. Even though medical practices cannot compete with most hospitals regarding wages, an RN will demand equitable pay with hospital nurses. The attraction of not working weekends or holidays can be sold only so far. If an RN is hired by the practice, it should plan on paying more that it would for an LPN or a UAP. Based on the many surveys taken locally and nationally, in both hospital nursing and office nursing, most RNs prefer office nursing.

The pay difference stimulates the need for all team members to be used effectively to the top of their capabilities and licensure. It may be cost effective to hire an RN if she/he will be complementing the role of the provider and allow them to expand their reach. Their pay could easily be justified if it allows the physician to see more patients and/or provide better care to obtain better reimbursement.

Chapter 3

Nursing Functions in a Medical Practice

In establishing the right staff for any medical clinic, the first step is to determine what functions the staff currently perform. Numerous tasks fall under the "clinical" umbrella. However, some of these tasks often overlap with front office or business office duties. The nurse may determine coding for laboratory tests, or the front office may gather reports for the visit or place patients in rooms. Regardless of who performs what function, the front office and business office must work with nursing to make the practice run smoothly. Likewise, nursing must work with other departments—no department can function without the other. Clinical and administrative aspects of any office are very interdependent.

Nursing is so broad that it would be impossible to list all its functions for primary care, let alone each clinical specialty. Therefore, a brief overview of nursing care functions is given, along with how these tasks differ from specialty to specialty. The use of licensed vs. non-licensed staff is also explored further. A more in-depth look at nursing functions as they relate to efficiency is provided in Chapter 5.

MAIN NURSING FUNCTIONS

Clinical and nursing functions may often overlap in a medical office. For the purposes of this book, nursing functions are defined as any task performed by nursing staff in a medical practice. Clinical functions are broader and encompasses all patient care activities, including those of physician, provider and ancillary staff. Some debate about who should perform these functions will almost certainly occur in the practice, but essentially, in most practices, nursing is responsible for phone management, patient flow, nursing procedures, pharmacology, supplies, and community resources. As medical offices move to a more value-based approach to care (i.e. focused on the quality of care provided versus quantity of care provided), nursing has broadened its functionality to include care coordination, population health, and care management. A brief explanation of each function follows, and a more detailed exploration of each is presented in later chapters.

PHONE MANAGEMENT

One of the more time-consuming tasks for both reception and nursing staff in many practices is managing telephone communications. Reasons for phone calls vary depending on the specialty. Patients call the practice to ask questions about medications, treatments, test results, symptoms, and many other concerns. Phone calls vary in length and complexity and require follow-up work. Handling phone calls coming into the practice in large part involves the nursing staff, and thus good phone management requires a significant amount of nursing time. Quantifying the volume and type of phone calls can assist in identifying both staffing and process needs.

The term phone triage is often used when discussing phone management. Phone management is related to distributing the phone call effectively, such as the receptionist answering the phone and determining if the call relates to nursing. Unlicensed clinical staff are often used for secondary phone management, such as determining whether the patient's issue can be managed over the phone or if it requires a visit. Often, an experienced unlicensed clinical staff member can give simple nursing advice per protocol and/or past experience.

True phone triage is a clinical function and often requires the skills and expertise of licensed nursing staff as it relates to clinical decision making. Licensed nurses determine the patient's need and plan of action, oftentimes using nursing judgement to dispense advice to the patient. Clinical decision making allows the nurse to assess the information given and choose a course of action.

PATIENT FLOW

Patient flow is a broad term used to define the movement of patients through the practice. Patient flow begins and is greatly affected by the preparation of the patient's chart—either electronic or paper. Chart preparation may be done at patient arrival, or it may be completed several days before the patient arrives in a process called pre-visit planning. Pre-visit planning is essential for the physician to provide the most appropriate care to the patient and is often done for all patients, especially those with a chronic illness such as diabetes, hypertension, or cancer. Consider a patient visit in an oncologist's office: without the patient's mammogram or surgical pathology report already available in the chart, how would the oncologist determine the treatment plan at the time of the visit? Adequate pre-visit planning helps avoid a wasted visit for both the oncologist and the patient.

Pre-visit planning includes looking at the medical record to determine if there is a need to do anything prior to the physician visit, such as:

- Gather any hospitalizations or emergency room visit information such as labs or imaging, consults, discharge summaries or other correspondence,

- Obtain any reports from referrals to specialists of community agencies such as home health,

- Complete any evidence-based guideline chronic disease protocols (i.e. for diabetes, A1c blood test every three months or ophthalmology exam once a year) or preventive care such as cancer screening (i.e. colorectal screening every 10 years or mammogram every one to two years) or immunizations (i.e. influenza or childhood vaccinations), and/or

- Ensure that all tests ordered from last visit or prior to this visit are on the medical record.

Rooming patients—ushering them to an examination room and performing preliminary tasks in preparation for the physician's visit—is a major part of patient flow. The goal in most clinics is to keep the physicians or midlevel providers moving from one patient to the next with minimal lag time. The typical process of assigning patients to a room is as follows: The patient is brought to an examination room, where the nursing staff member takes a brief history or documents the chief complaint, takes vital signs, and ensures chart preparation and any needed testing are completed. Nursing staff may also gather social, surgical, or medical history. They may also ask questions about preventive or chronic disease protocols. Nursing also prepares the patient for the exam, which may include asking him or her to undress, setting out supplies, or obtaining consents for treatment.

The patient flow process is usually dictated by the physician and can vary widely by practice. Specialty physicians such as ophthalmologists or podiatrists are not as concerned about vital signs, for example, whereas primary care physicians may require them. Variations in the history-taking function may include nursing staff collecting the history, the patient completing the history with nursing overview, or the physician interviewing and completing the history.

One skill that is essential for good patient flow is the ability to make each patient comfortable while at the same time keeping the physician moving efficiently from one patient to the next. An example from one practice demonstrates a less than optimal ability to control patient flow: The physician had an assistant who was very personable. He loved to chat with patients and wanted to make them comfortable prior to the physician entering the room. However, the physician often had to wait for him to complete his chat with the patients. The assistant did not have the ability to break away from the patients and allow the physician to keep moving. Nursing's role in this situation is to seek information from the patient in a quick and friendly manner.

As the physician sees patients, the nursing staff may be asked to provide assistance to the physician during a procedure or an exam. For example, male physicians often request that a female nurse or assistant be in the room for breast or pelvic exams. Procedures such as biopsies or excisions require the assistance of nursing staff.

Communication with the front desk is vital to good patient flow, and timing is critical. If the nurse has five minutes to room a patient before he or she is needed to assist the physician with a procedure, the nurse and the front desk staff need to communicate effectively to ensure that the next patient is ready to be seen. Communication needs between nursing and the front desk include:

- Notification of patient arrival;
- Retrieval of the paper or electronic chart;
- Management of unexpected circumstances such as the arrival of walk-in patients;
- Updates on scheduling; and
- Physician wait time.

Sometimes in practices, conflict arises between nursing and front desk staff—nursing staff complain about the front desk, and the front desk staff complain about nursing. If patient flow is a problem in your practice, look at the relationship and communication level between the front desk and nursing. It is critical for both to work together.

Communication with the physician or provider is also vital in making patient flow work well. Communication needs between physicians and nursing include:

- Notification of patient readiness;
- Requirement for nursing assistance; and
- The need for follow-up nursing care.

Often communication can be streamlined through the use of a "huddle" or simple meeting prior to starting the day or session. The huddle is a quick conversation about patients on the schedule for that session or day and last no more than 5 minutes. Pre-visit planning plays a key part in the huddle, since the nursing staff will have a good look at what patient needs are and can quickly inform the provider. Attendees should include the provider, the roomer and any other key members of the team affecting the workflow for that session or day.

Another patient flow reality are visits from pharmacological company representatives (i.e., drug reps) with the physician during office hours. Physician preferences vary on this issue, depending on the need for samples, and other factors and each practice will handle this differently.

After the physician sees the patient, orders and follow-up will determine the next step in patient flow. If no orders are given, the patient may leave. Depending on the practice, either nursing or the physician may dismiss the patient. The final part of patient flow is seeing the patient out of the practice or back to the front desk.

NURSING PROCEDURES

Before, during, or after the physician's visit with the patient, the nursing staff may be asked to perform any number of procedures. The most notable fall in the area of medication administration. Other responsibilities may include wound or dressing care, staple or suture removal, irrigations, or testing procedures such as electrocardiograms (EKGs) or spirometry.

In addition, an important nursing function is patient education. Although physicians educate patients, often patients need reinforcement or time to ask more questions. For example, in a surgeon's office, the surgeon may explain to the patient the surgery, risks, complications, and indications. When the surgeon leaves the room, however, the patient often asks the nursing staff one or more questions he or she was uncomfortable asking the surgeon, or seeks clarification on what he or she has just heard. This may be the case in many other situations. Patient education, if done well at the time of the visit, reduces calls after the visit; if done poorly or incompletely can increase phone volume or cause the practice to lose patients.

Education is a primary objective of any office visit, even during a procedure. With today's declining reimbursements, physicians must see more patients to compensate and thus have less time to explain and teach the patient. More and more often, it is a nursing responsibility to make sure the patient is well informed about his or her condition. Education can be given in person, through handouts, through the patient portal, or through recommended websites. This will vary dependent upon the practice population. Oftentimes, a quick one-page summary of the day's visit, such as a clinical summary, is given to the patient or sent through a patient portal, so the patient can review the information at their leisure or share with family.

At times, patients come to the clinic to see the nurse rather than the physician for such reasons as blood pressure checks, medication samples, injections, dressing changes, and immunizations. These visits, too, affect patient flow, because chart preparation, rooming, and overall patient flow still must be taken into account.

MEDICATION MANAGEMENT

Pharmacological management is a large part of any nursing staff's responsibilities, and it begins with rooming patients. Medical care often includes the use of medication in the treatment plan. Without knowledge of the patient's past and present medication history, the physician might not be able to properly treat the patient and, in some cases, may harm the patient (e.g., patients using blood-thinning medication cannot undergo procedures without adjusting or stopping the dose).

Medication reconciliation is the process of identifying the most complete and accurate list of medications a patient is taking, reviewing each medication for indication, effectiveness and possible adverse events, and resolving any discrepancies between other sources of medication listed. The purpose of reconciliation is to avoid errors of transcription, omission, duplication of therapy, drug-drug interactions, and/or drug-disease interactions.

Medication reconciliation often requires medical or clinical decision making because it entails the review of medications, their indication, effectiveness, and possible adverse events. It often requires the skills and expertise of a physician, pharmacist or an experienced nurse. Medication review is a better description of the role the MA may take in the practice.

The administering of medications by nursing staff can occur in numerous ways: injection, inhalation, intravenous infusion, or mouth or skin.

Nursing staff are also charged with teaching patients about medications. Medication education leads to medication compliance and adherence. If patients understand why they are on the medication, what the side effects are, and what outcome is to be achieved, they will be more likely to adhere to the medication treatment as prescribed. Many electronic medical records allow the provider to see which prescriptions have been filled to determine medication adherence. A great proportion of hospital admissions are the result of poor medication compliance.

Finally, dispensing sample medications may fall under nursing's responsibility. The nursing staff follow physician instructions regarding what samples to provide to patients.

SUPPLY MANAGEMENT

Some medical supplies are used during most office visits. Nursing staff is responsible for maintaining supplies in the exam rooms, procedure rooms, and stockroom.

CARE MANAGEMENT

Medical offices, especially primary care, may need to supplement their management of chronically ill patients with care management. Care management is providing complementary one-on-one chronic disease care and care coordination to those patients who are at high risk for hospitalizations or emergency room visits. Population health can help identify those patients in need of more assistance. The goal is to reduce utilization and to increase quality of care for those patients. A registered nurse is often used in this role because of the need for clinical decision making. The "care manager" complements the chronic disease care provided by the care team (i.e. provider and medical assistant) for those patients who are outside of the normal parameters, such as diabetics who have high Hgb A1c levels or oncology patients with multiple illnesses that are complicating their cancer care.

The practice typically determines criteria for care management, such as multiple hospital stays, multiple emergency room visits, eight or more medications, two or more chronic diseases including psychiatric disease, frequent physician office visits, patients outside normal parameters.

Office staff and providers may struggle with how to integrate this new team member into their team and need clarity on the role and expectations. Inviting them to team huddles, or establishing communication channels are often effective.

ONE-ON-ONE CHRONIC DISEASE CARE

Many times patients have a new diagnosis or an exacerbation of their current disease that may lead to hospitalization. An RN, health coach or health educator may be asked to assist them in returning them back to normal functioning. Perhaps they need education on their disease, self-care management or how to recognize symptoms that lead to trouble. A care plan is created to guide the care and to communicate to all team members. The care plan includes objective and subjective assessment and reason for extra assistance. Collaborative goal setting with the patient and Interventions are also included. Once the patient has stabilized, the extra assistance is no longer needed and the patient returns to the care team for management.

POPULATION HEALTH

Managing the entire panel of patients in a medical office or for a specific physician or provider, requires population health strategies. Population health allows the practice to understand their patients better. For instance, a practice might have 80% of their patients who are over 65. This can help guide programs and/or education efforts for staff and patients. Population health is used to better understand the entire panel, chronic disease populations and preventive health. If a physician knows 20% of his population has a diagnosis of hypertension and only 40% are adequately controlled with a blood pressure under 140/90, he can take action on getting those patients better controlled. If a physician knows he has 40% teenagers in his panel of patients and that 50% of them smoke, then he can set up programs to help prevent smoking and/or engage his team in helping those smokers quit.

As more practices have started using electronic medical records, population health has become more manageable and data more available to analyze. Practices need to ensure that data is entered correctly, that reports are run and analyzed, and that actions are taken and evaluated for effectiveness.

CARE COORDINATION

Care coordination encompasses everything that is done outside a medical office. Patients sometimes have difficulty navigating health care and need someone to guide them through the maze of other health care providers and community resources. Other health care providers include hospitals, nursing homes, home health agencies, rehabilitation facilities, outpatient therapy providers, other physicians, etc. Community resources can encompass any other needs such as transportation, help with groceries, senior centers, churches, medical equipment providers, etc.

Oftentimes, a practice will provide care coordination services with a navigator or care coordinator who helps guide the patient through this maze by making referrals and following up on hospitalizations and specialist referrals. This role can easily be assumed by an unlicensed clinical or clerical staff member who can assist patients. But if combined with chronic disease clinical decision making, it would require the licensure of a nurse.

OTHER DUTIES

"Other duties" is the catchall category for all the various additional responsibilities that fall to nursing in coordinating the patient's care. Working with community resources constitutes a significant part of this category and includes the following:

- Insurance companies and third-party payers. Pre-certification can be the responsibility of the nursing staff, and hospital stays can include nursing's responsibility for case management services.

- Diagnostic testing follow-up. Any test ordered by the physician should be tracked to ensure the results are received and shared with the patient. If no tracking is done, the test result may never reach the clinic.

- Coding for pre-certification, diagnostic testing, or procedures.

- Prescription discount programs requiring extensive completion of forms.

- Completing Family Medical Leave Act or disability paperwork.

- Quality-of-care standards, including ensuring appropriate and safe care is provided to patients and then, often, reporting this information.

- Patient satisfaction.

- Clinical trial management. Understanding criteria and requirements helps guide patients to research studies performed in or out of the office.

The tasks on the above list, though not inclusive, can be taken on by different departments as the clinic size increases.

Because the list of possible nursing functions is lengthy, it is very important to identify which nursing functions are being used in the clinic.

DIFFERING FUNCTIONS DEPEND ON SPECIALITY

Nursing functions will change in complexity and need depending on the specialty. In primary care practices—family practice, internal medicine, pediatrics—the patients are usually long term and the primary care practice provider becomes a coordinator of care. Some specialist providers—surgery; orthopedics; gastro-enterology; hospitalist; allergist; otolaryngology (ears, nose, and throat); dermatology; etc.—have short-term involvement with the patient. They see the patient, fix what is wrong, and then never see the patient again or see him or her on a very infrequent basis. Some specialist providers—cardiology, rheumatology, pulmonology, oncology, etc.—can become more like primary care providers to an extent. They consult on a specific condition and take over the care of that condition for the long term.

The discussion that follows makes some assumptions regarding separating primary care from specialty practices. However, as stated above, this distinction is not always clear and should be weighed carefully in making any staffing decisions.

Primary care providers have a heavy workload for nursing staff, with extensive phone management, medication management, and community resource management. Family practice and pediatrics may experience additional stress because of the frequency of vaccinations in such practices. Primary care physicians are often communicating regularly with specialist providers and coordinating the care of patients with those providers. For instance, after the hospitalist has released the patient from the hospital, he or she turns the care over to the primary care physician. A change in medication or treatment could have occurred during hospitalization that now has to be managed by the primary care physician. Communication and documentation of that hospital visit are crucial in continuing patient care.

In contrast, specialty provider nursing staff encounter less phone management, less medication management, and less community resource management than do those in primary care, family practice, or pediatrics. However, other skills and functions likely replace the aforementioned functions. In a surgical practice, nursing may be responsible for pre-certification and assisting with procedures instead of phone triage. An oncology office might have a mixture of both—heavy phone and medication management as well as a high level of procedures, such as injections or intravenous (IV) therapy.

USE OF LICENSED OR NON-LICENSED NURSING STAFF

As practices move towards team-based care, decisions on whether to use licensed staff or unlicensed staff will arise. So the question becomes, what functions really require the expertise of a registered nurse, and what functions can be delegated to other nursing staff?

Delegation to non-licensed nursing staff is covered in more depth in Chapter 6. For the purposes of this discussion, consider the following points.

Competency has to be established prior to delegation. If a medical assistant is assigned to the task of rooming patients—taking vital signs, conducting a medication review, taking the medical history, preparing the chart—make sure, by watching and reviewing, that he or she is competent to perform that task. Do not just take the assistant's word that he or she has adequate training and skills.

Nurses say that even the simplest task—rooming patients—is crucial to a good office visit. Talking with the patient gives the RN a good sense of the patient's concerns. The nurse may be able to streamline the patient's questions prior to the physician's visit. Taking vital signs and history may signal a problem to an RN that can be brought to the physician's attention—a problem that may be overlooked by the non-licensed staff. Even verifying medications can be critical, as accuracy is essential. Sometimes, however, a trade-off must be made between cost and quality of staff.

Front office staff can assist nursing immeasurably. In a pinch, they can assist with medication list verification, rooming patients, or supply management. The more experienced the front office staff, the bigger the difference they can make.

NURSING TASKS NOT REQUIRING LICENSED STAFF

If properly trained, the non-licensed nursing staff can take responsibility for the following:

- Rooming patients—including chart preparation, pre-visit planning, taking vital signs, taking history
- Assisting physician with procedures
- Performing testing procedures—EKG, spirometry, etc.
- Preparing medication lists
- Acquiring drug samples
- Stocking rooms
- Managing supplies
- Performing insurance precertification, follow-up
- Preparing referrals to specialists
- Communicating with community resources
- Performing simple nursing procedures—removing sutures, changing dressings, etc.

With intense training and competency validation, unlicensed assistive personnel can help with the following:

- Injections—allergy, subcutaneous, intramuscular (requires extensive
- instruction)
- Tuberculosis testing
- Vaccinations
- Wound care
- Medication refills
- Telephone duty—answering the phones and taking messages

Nursing Tasks Requiring Licensed Staff

Using a licensed nurse is appropriate in certain situations, such as:

1. Phone triage, in which the nurse gives the patient advice or nursing care over the phone, reviews symptoms, or provides teaching;

2. Administration of chemotherapy, IV medications, or complex injections; and

3. Complex patient education requiring analysis of particular patient situations.

The key factor in all of these tasks is the nurse's ability to use clinical decision making. The competency and training needed to answer phone calls and triage those calls are vastly different from those required to just take messages and allow the physician to answer the calls. An unlicensed assistive person may be able to function in the latter role, but not the former.

The argument that an experienced medical assistant or nursing assistant can perform phone triage or nursing duties may be valid in specific situations. However, a nurse is required to take numerous courses to prepare him or her to provide nursing care, including anatomy and physiology, nursing process, and medication administration. A medical assistant or nursing assistant has not had that preparation, regardless of how long he or she has worked in the field. In short, assistants cannot make the same decisions as nurses because they have not received the education necessary to support their decision making.

In some specialties, little need exists for complete phone triage, patient education, or other highly technical skills. Using an unlicensed person to perform these duties may be appropriate if he or she knows his or her limitations.

The bottom line is to ensure that all staff members work to the top of their capability and licensure. Having a robust discussion about roles and tasks is a good step for any practice to take.

Chapter 4

Staff Accountability

Every situation is unique. Nursing should be measured by keeping in mind the nature of nursing itself. Nursing is about taking care of patients. Achieving target numbers is not meaningful if patients are not cared for effectively.

Nursing has struggled with staffing for many years. Pick up any nursing magazine and you will see that hospital staffing issues top the headlines. Staffing approaches in hospitals have become more refined, but the human element remains the most important factor in their application. If your mother is a patient at the hospital, you are not concerned about how much her care costs. The same concept applies to the physician's office. Your concern is that the nursing staff takes care of her.

Types of productivity measures are explained in this chapter. Ultimately, after the numbers have been tabulated, the manager should carefully review the data in the context of patient care to make sure that, whatever adjustments are made, the essence of nursing care remains a big part of the practice.

MEASURES

There are numerous measures that can be used to determine accountability for patient care. Quality measures are often used to determine the health of the population served. For example, a pediatric practice can be measured on the number of children who have been immunized or the percent of children who have had their well-child checks. This is more of a team measure rather than an individual measure, since the patient touches many team members that might have a part in completing this measure. Quality measures can give us a good picture of how the team is functioning as a whole.

Another measure that might be used to determine accountability of the team is a financial benchmark. The total cost of care for a panel of patients might be one benchmark, or utilization costs related to hospitalization or use of services might be another. Although certain members of the team have greater roles in the cost of care, other team members can influence this as well. For example, a physician makes the decision as to whether the patient should be hospitalized, but the phone operator or scheduler controls the gateway for patients to access the physician or be sent to the emergency room.

Efficiency measures are often used to quantify accountability for patient care. Metrics, such as completing the patient assessment at rooming with vital signs, questions about smoking or advanced directives give us some measure of how the team functions collectively and individually. Measuring access to care such as continuity (i.e. seeing the same provider) and ability to see same-day patients also give us some measure of how the team functions.

When we look at the nursing role, one of the first questions to answer when looking at productivity is what exactly can be measured. One measure should never be used exclusively to determine staffing or productivity. If two to three measures are pointing in one direction, then that direction should be explored further before making any staffing decisions.

Measures discussed in this section include nursing productivity measures, such as

- visits;
- phone calls;
- procedures performed; and
- time study.

Any of these approaches will give the manager data to help determine productivity of the physicians and, subsequently, of nursing. Nursing productivity is often tied to physician productivity in some way because their efforts in providing patient care are so closely aligned.

In performing staffing analysis, practice management and electronic medical record reports are helpful but somewhat limited. Time is required to gather and analyze the data. Some electronic systems can provide raw data, but using those data may require manually counting specific data points. For instance, the practice management system may generate schedules but not visit times in aggregate to measure peak scheduling times.

Another point to bear in mind when collecting data is that the data are only as good as the person collecting them. One way to ensure accurate data collection is to clearly define what data to collect and where it should be entered into the medical record, followed by watching as the calculations and observations take place. Another method is to collect enough data over a long enough period of time to add validity to the results. Stressing the importance of the data collection is the first step in collecting accurate data, and involving staff in the process also assists in collection efforts.

Examples of data collection and analysis follow. Sometimes, identifying staffing inefficiencies is easy just by looking at one graph, and acting on the discovery may be straightforward. However, caution is advised when making a staffing decision based on one view. In Chapter 7, data collection is further analyzed to determine staffing needs.

VISITS

One of the most visual representations of activity in any practice is its number and type of visits. A table with a visual representation of the volume of visits by day of the month gives a clear picture of the practice activity over a month's time. The appointment schedule can be used to gather this information, as it documents the date, time, physician, and appointment type. In analyzing visit data, no-show patients should be excluded from the analysis.

First we consider a basic analysis of visits per provider per day. The example used here is a hospital-owned family practice clinic with six physicians. After interviews were conducted with nursing staff, it became apparent that a staff conflict existed. Some nursing staff felt they were working harder than others because their own physicians were busier. In addition to determining how to reduce conflict, the manager of the practice was also reviewing a request by nursing staff that each be allowed a half day off during the week. Appointment schedules were examined and visits were tabulated by physician, by day for several months' time. **Exhibit 4.1** displays the resulting data.

This table represents two weeks out of the entire time considered. Keep in mind that, for a complete analysis, totals for two to three months provide a better picture than this short period because they tend to balance out variations in physicians' schedules. Be aware also that this table is very simple. Changes can be made depending on the needs of the practice, such as adding average visit per day by physician or average visits per week by physician.

EXHIBIT 4.1 Visits per Day

	M	Tu	W	Th	F	M	Tu	W	Th	F	Total
Doctor 1	20	25	22	27	15	15	18	22	25	20	209
Doctor 2	39	31	16	33	37	40	31	19	34	37	317
Doctor 3	16	17	15	15	15	16	17	15	15	15	156
Doctor 4	22	28	32	29	20	20	29	30	28	22	260
Doctor 5	21	15	21	22	25	25	22	21	16	22	210
Doctor 6	40	16	35	38	31	45	20	35	40	25	325
Total	158	132	141	164	143	161	137	142	158	141	

These data reveal that Doctor 2 and Doctor 6 are consistently the busiest in the practice, and Doctor 3's productivity is below that of the others. For example, Doctor 6 likely works only a half day on Tuesdays. Mondays and Thursdays appear to be the busiest days in the practice—an apparent trend that can be verified with further analysis. Some variation is also seen by physician in the physicians' daily schedules. The charts in **Exhibits 4.2** and **4.3** can assist in finding out which are the busiest days of the week and what variations occur during each day. (The data in these exhibits were collected from the same schedules and tabulated to add more clarity at the end of the report used for **Exhibit 4.1**.)

EXHIBIT 4.2 Visits on the Busiest Days

	M	Tu	W	Th	F
Week 1	158	132	141	164	135
Week 2	160	135	145	165	130
Week 3	165	120	125	170	140
Week 4	180	111	120	158	145
Week 5	150	122	135	165	135
Total	813	620	666	822	685
Average	163	124	133	164	137

According to the results shown in **Exhibit 4.2**, Mondays and Thursdays are the busiest days in the practice on average, and Tuesdays, Wednesdays, and Fridays are slower days. Once again, it is advisable to look at several months' data to validate these findings.

Breaking down the individual physician variation during the day is the next step (see **Exhibit 4.3**). The data can be analyzed by hour, by morning, or by afternoon, depending on what questions need answers relating to visits per day per provider. In this example, several physicians have afternoons or mornings off, so looking at staffing needs by half day lends a better understanding of the relevant trends. As before, the data are collected from the daily appointment schedule.

EXHIBIT 4.3 Visits: Variation during the Day										
	M		**Tu**		**W**		**Th**		**F**	
	a.m.	p.m.	a.m.	p.m.	a.m.	p.m.	a.m.	p.m.	a.m.	p.m.	Total
Doctor 1	10	10	10	10	10	10	10	10	10	10	100
Doctor 2	15		15	15	15	15	15	15	15	15	135
Doctor 3	20		20	20	20	20	20	20	20	20	180
Doctor 4	10	15	10	15	10		15	10	15	10	110
Doctor 5	20	15	20	10	15		15	20	20	10	145
Doctor 6	10	15	10	15	10	15		15	20	15	125
Total	85	55	85	85	80	60	75	90	100	80	

This example shows that on Monday and Wednesday afternoons, the practice is not as busy because two physicians are out of the office. This information may represent an opportunity to give several nursing staff members those afternoons off. The analysis would be more significant in a specialist office in which the physician may be out of the office for periods of time. To explore such a scenario, consider the example in **Exhibit 4.4** of a three-physician surgeon practice.

Doctor 1 is in surgery every morning, while Doctors 2 and 3 have varying surgery schedules. Staffing for the office could fluctuate depending on other needs of the practice. In this example, one full-time nurse, with a part-time nurse on Tuesday, Thursday, and Friday afternoons, could probably manage this office.

EXHIBIT 4.4 Visits to Specialist

	M a.m.	M p.m.	Tu a.m.	Tu p.m.	W a.m.	W p.m.	Th a.m.	Th p.m.	F a.m.	F p.m.
Doctor 1		10		10		10		10		10
Doctor 2			15	15				15		15
Doctor 3				20		20	20	20		20
Total	0	10	15	45	0	30	20	45	0	45

As you can see, determining staffing needs for a particular office begins with a visual display of the data related to physician visits. Variations of the above examples are limitless. For example, productivity projections can be used when adding another provider. The practice manager can project the days and visit numbers for the new provider and then determine staffing needs as a whole. Taking the example a step further, if the practice has a less productive physician, he or she can share staff with the new provider.

EXHIBIT 4.5 Visits by Type

	M	Tu	W	Th	F	M	Tu	W	Th	F	Total
Doctor 1	16	17	15	15	15	16	17	15	15	15	156
New	1	5	1	2	2	2	3	1	1	1	19
Establish	14	12	14	13	12	13	13	14	13	14	132
Proc	1	0	0	0	1	1	1	0	1	0	5
Doctor 2	40	16	35	38	31	45	20	35	40	25	325
New	10	8	7	11	6	15	8	7	6	11	89
Establish	26	4	25	26	25	27	10	24	31	12	210
Proc	4	4	3	1	0	3	2	4	3	2	26

Another component of the visit study is type of visits performed. The example that follows depicts a two pediatric physician practice. Such a study can answer several questions about staffing, as discussed below. Here, Doctor 1 is in the latter part of his career and therefore sees fewer total patients and takes on fewer new patients. Doctor 2 is younger, and his practice is growing rapidly. The first row in **Exhibit 4.5,** labeled "Doctor 1," shows total visits for that day. The visit totals are then broken down by category (new, established, or procedure) and appear in the rows below the doctors' totals. If desired, weekly totals can be added and then tabulated as well. Visit schedules were used to obtain the data for this study.

Doctor 1, who is not as productive as Doctor 2, is also not seeing as many new patients or performing as many procedures as Doctor 2. Doctor 2 thus needs more staffing because he almost doubles the production of Doctor 1 and because he sees more new patients and performs more procedures, all of which involve more nursing time. As with earlier examples, analyzing several months' worth of data will validate (or invalidate) the findings.

Another way to look at visits by physician to determine staffing is on a monthly basis with average visits per day. Although any practice will experience busy days and not-so-busy days, determining average visits by day can help gauge staffing over the long term. This average evens out the ebbs and flows of visit volume and reveals changes in the practice over time. Once compiled, the data might look like those shown in **Exhibit 4.6**.

EXHIBIT 4.6 Average Visits by Day			
	Doctor 1	Doctor 2	Doctor 3
Days in Office Available for Visits			
April	14.5	17.5	18.5
May	14.5	16.0	15.5
June	16.5	15.5	14.0
July	13.0	15.0	14.5
Total	58.5	64.0	62.5
Office Visits			
April	231	671	293
May	247	549	206
June	236	546	187
July	241	600	211
Total	955	2,366	897
Average Visits per Day Total	16.32	36.97	14.35

The average visit per day is calculated by dividing total visits by average days in the office. Doctor 2 is much busier than Doctors 1 and 3, which may indicate she needs more staffing. This type of analysis provides a bird's eye view of the practice as a whole. One variation of such a study for a family practice can show nursing home visits and minor surgery visits in addition to total visits. Nursing visits can also be broken down to determine the types of these visits experienced in an average month.

A final approach to viewing visit totals is simply to look at the raw numbers of total provider visits as a percentage of total visits. This type of analysis helps pinpoint the proportion of resources each physician requires. Relative value units can also be used to tabulate physicians' proportional use of resources. The table shown in **Exhibit 4.7** examines three doctors' visit totals over four months. Doctors 1 and 2 appear to require more resources to care for their patients than does Doctor 3.

EXHIBIT 4.7 Visits as a Percentage of Resources						
	May	June	July	August	Total	%
Doctor 1	255	256	262	263	1,036	36
Doctor 2	304	336	218	213	1,071	37
Doctor 3	213	220	189	170	792	27
					2,899	

PHONE CALLS

Telephone calls can monopolize nursing time, especially in primary care practices, so analysis of nurses' phone duty volume provides a good productivity measure. Phone calls vary in length depending on the reason for the call. One interesting data set for telephone usage volume is the total number of calls received and a breakdown of reasons for the calls. Such a study requires staff to document every phone call made to the practice. To add validity to the study, a phone system report or the phone attendant should also be involved, documenting each phone call to the practice and tracking the numbers by department. A simple tabulating sheet (see **Exhibit 4.8**) can be created for the phone attendant.

Tracking phone call volume in the nursing area begins with identifying the major reasons for the calls. **Exhibit 4.9** shows an expanded nursing call log.

Why are the reasons important? After looking at the results, a manager may see that nursing is spending a considerable amount of time making or rescheduling appointments. Are the phone calls being routed appropriately? Is the phone attendant asking enough questions before routing the call? Similarly, if questions about medications constitute a large percentage of phone call queries, can a procedure be established to make sure the medications are fully understood by patients during the appointment, eliminating the need for a follow-up phone call? The office may need to develop medication teaching processes, complete with patient education materials, to fully educate the patient at the appointment. If phone calls regarding test results are high in volume, can the practice better use the nurse's time by setting up an automated system for test result reporting?

EXHIBIT 4.8 Example of a Phone Call Log: Practice			
Date and Time	Billing	Nursing	Other

Nursing staff should be given instructions to document time of day and to place a check mark in the box that best describes the nature of the call. In addition to tracking calls coming into the office, outgoing calls may be tracked using a reverse study if nursing is found to be making a high volume of calls out. In this approach, have the nursing staff mark a chart similar to that shown in **Exhibit 4.9** indicating the reason for every outgoing call to a patient.

EXHIBIT 4.9 Example of a Phone Call Log: Nursing

Date and Time	Medication	Symptom Control	Test Results	Appointments	Other

After tabulating the results, you should be able to identify call volume as a whole and by time of day. An example of a completed phone log is shown in **Exhibit 4.10**.

EXHIBIT 4.10 Phone Call Log by Hour

Phone Calls for July	M	Tu	W	Th	F	Total	%
Before 9 a.m.	32	17	16	14	14	93	15
9-10 a.m.	27	19	18	15	17	96	16
10-11 a.m.	27	16	16	12	13	84	14
11-12 noon	27	11	6	10	8	62	10
12-1 p.m.	9	13	14	9	11	56	9
1-2 p.m.	6	8	4	5	5	28	5
2-3 p.m.	13	14	15	8	15	65	11
3-4 p.m.	9	10	18	15	9	61	10
4-5 p.m.	15	11	11	14	13	64	11
Total	165	119	118	102	105	609	
Percentage	27%	20%	19%	17%	17%		

Complete the charts each day for more than one week, and then compile the results. The data from these logs can be broken down by hour, by day, and by physician to help determine staffing needs. In the scenario shown in **Exhibit 4.10**, a large phone call volume is experienced at the beginning of the day, with 45 percent of calls occurring before 11 a.m. Is the practice staffed for that call volume? Between 12 p.m. and 2 p.m., the call volume is much lower. Are the nursing staff taking lunch during that time?

The answer to the latter question for one practice was that nursing staff were too busy with phone calls at lunchtime to take lunch. A phone study for calls in and calls out at this practice revealed the nursing staff were making all of their return phone calls at lunchtime. If this situation occurs at your practice, consider having another staff member assist nursing with calls first thing in the morning so they can be caught up by lunch.

Exhibit 4.10 also shows that call volume is heavier on Monday, the first day following the weekend on which patients can call the office for assistance. Perhaps more staff are needed to answer phone calls on Monday than during the rest of the week.

The results of a phone call volume study can also be broken down by physician and, subsequently, by nurse (see **Exhibit 4.11**). The phone calls can also be broken down by type of call.

EXHIBIT 4.11 Phone Calls Divided by Nurse						
	Total	Medication	Symptom Control	Test Results	Appointments	Other
Nurse 1						
Nurse 2						
Nurse 3						

Practice patterns emerge to demonstrate phone call demographics. This information can be used in the overall nursing productivity picture.

PROCEDURES PERFORMED

Tracking procedures performed by nursing staff can help determine staffing needs. One example of this approach is seen in a family practice clinic that assigns a nurse to see walk-in patients for the day. The procedures performed by that nurse, including giving injections and vaccinations, taking blood pressures (BP), performing tuberculosis (TB) tests, and fulfilling requests for samples or other items, are quantified according to the method displayed in **Exhibit 4.12**.

EXHIBIT 4.12 Nursing Procedures

Function	M	Tu	W	Th	F
Weight check		1	3	2	1
TB test	1	3		2	
BP	5	10	11	6	2
O2 saturation	1	1		1	1
Vaccination	5	6	2	3	6
Suture removal			2		
Triage	4	4	2	3	1
Samples	3	3	2	3	3
Total	19	28	22	20	14

Overall, this table shows that nursing visits are evenly spread across the week. If it is found at your clinic that one day of the week typically sees an overwhelming volume of one procedure—blood pressure checks, for example—the physicians can be asked to guide patients to visit on different days to spread them out.

A short time study (see the next section for more detailed information) can be conducted to quantify the average time needed to handle any one of these types of visits. For instance, if a nurse takes, on average, 10 minutes to perform a blood pressure check on a patient—bringing the patient back to a room, performing the blood pressure check, talking to the patient, recording results—then he or she will spend 100 minutes, or 1 hour and 40 minutes, taking 10 blood pressures. In this way, information about the total time needed to staff a walk-in nurse is provided. Time studies are especially applicable to oncology clinics—an area of practice that sees many nursing visits. Nursing staff's time spent performing chemotherapy, injections, rooming patients, and other duties can be quantified as described above to determine staffing needs.

TIME STUDY

As indicated in the previous section, time studies can be used to evaluate further staffing and operational needs. The following two time studies were undertaken to answer questions surrounding these needs. Time study 1 looks at the best use of time in patient flow through the practice. Time study 2 considers staffing hours in relation to actual clinical time spent.

TIME STUDY 1

In the practice that undertook this study, a recurring theme of long patient visit times developed when areas of concern were explored among staff and physicians. Nursing staff stated that the front desk personnel were not getting the patients signed in upon arrival quickly enough and the physicians were not seeing the patients as soon as they were placed in rooms. The front desk stated that the nursing staff did not pick up the visiting patients' charts quickly enough, and therefore, the patients sat in the waiting room too long. The physicians stated that the nursing staff were sitting at the nursing station while their patients waited in the waiting room.

Many factors can cause a delay. To pinpoint problem areas in this practice, a time study was conducted. This study required cooperation of all staff, and because concern was expressed by all staff, complete buy-in was achieved. At each of the following stages, the person who interacted with the patient noted the time on a time ticket (see **Exhibit 4.13**), which was attached to the charge ticket (also known as a fee ticket or routing slip) that was placed with each chart when the patient checked in:

- The patient checks in at the front desk.

- The front desk places the chart at the window for nurse pickup.

- The nurse picks up the chart, takes the patient into the examination room, and turns on a light to notify the physician that a patient is ready to be seen.

- The physician enters the room.

Recording these times on the charge ticket or setting up the electronic system to track time as the patient moves through the system can also be done. If an electronic medical record system is in place, it also may be used to track time. Once results are compiled, they can be tabulated as a whole and then by individual physician. The table shown in **Exhibit 4.14** displays the raw data from this time study.

EXHIBIT 4.13 Time Ticket

	Time-In
Check-in	
Chart in window	
Nurse takes chart	
Physician's light on	
Physician in room	

To make sense of these data, a second table is required that gives time value in minutes of time lost during the process (**Exhibit 4.15**). At this practice, the charge ticket was printed when the patient had finished with check-in. If the patient was not finished before the appointment time (positive number), it counted against the front desk and was added to the overall processing time. If the patient check-in was completed earlier than the appointment time (negative number), it was not counted in the total appointment time. In addition to the data collected for this study, a patient arrival time column may be added to clarify how much time it took the front desk to check in the patient. Another illuminating data set is the time the patient left the practice, which gives an overall visit time.

Referring back to **Exhibit 4.14**, patient 1's appointment was at 8:30 a.m., but check-in was not completed until 8:35, adding 5 minutes to the appointment time (seen in **Exhibit 4.15**). Nursing staff took another 9 minutes to pick up her chart, at 8:44 a.m. The nurse roomed the patient and turned on the physician's light at 8:50 a.m. The physician entered the room at 9:01 a.m., 11 minutes later. The total time spent on this process was 31 minutes.

EXHIBIT 4.14 Time Study 1 Raw Data					
Patient	Appointment Time	Check-in Time (Chart to Window)	Nurse Takes Chart from Window	Physician's Light On	Physician In Room
1	8:30 a.m.	8:35 a.m.	8:44 a.m.	8:50 a.m.	9.01 a.m.
2	8:45 a.m.	8.49 a.m.	8:55 a.m.	8:59 a.m.	9:00 a.m.
3	9:00 a.m.	8:52 a.m.	9:01 a.m.	9:07 a.m.	9:22 a.m.
4	9:00 a.m.	8:59 a.m.	9:00 a.m.	9:10 a.m.	9:13 a.m.
5	10:45 a.m.	10:29 a.m.	10:41 a.m.	10:50 a.m.	11:15 a.m.
6	9:00 a.m.	8:37 a.m.	8:40 a.m.	8:53 a.m.	9:10 a.m.
7	10:30 a.m.	10:28 a.m.	10:30 a.m.	10:35 a.m.	10:40 a.m.
8	11:00 a.m.	10:27 a.m.	10:41 a.m.	10:50 a.m.	10:55 a.m.
9	1:30 p.m.	1:30 p.m.	1:35 p.m.	1:40 p.m.	1:50 p.m.
10	1:30 p.m.	1:20 p.m.	1:35 p.m.	1:39 p.m.	1:45 p.m.
11	1:30 p.m.	1:28 p.m.	1:29 p.m.	1:45 p.m.	1:48 p.m.
12	1:30 p.m.	1:28 p.m.	1:33 p.m.	1:35 p.m.	1:40 p.m.
13	1:30 p.m.	1:35 p.m.	1:36 p.m.	1:44 p.m.	1:52 p.m.
14	2:00 p.m.	1:41 p.m.	1:45 p.m.	1:51 p.m.	2:17 p.m.
15	2:30 p.m.	2:31 p.m.	2:44 p.m.	2:46 p.m.	
16	2:45 p.m.	1:30 p.m.	1:38 p.m.	1:43 p.m.	1:45 p.m.
17	2:30 p.m.	2:15 p.m.	2:16 p.m.	2:20 p.m.	2:50 p.m.

Patient 6 checked in 23 minutes early, at 8:37, for a 9 a.m. appointment. The nurse took the chart at 8:40 a.m., roomed the patient, and was ready for the doctor at 8:53 a.m. The doctor did not come into the room until 9:10 a.m. This visit's process took 33 minutes.

As can be seen in **Exhibit 4.15**, some opportunities seem to be available for improvement. Overall processing time was more than 24 minutes per patient, not including check-in time unless it took place after the appointment time. On average, the nursing staff took six-and-a-half minutes to retrieve the checked-in patient's chart and six-and-a-half minutes to room the patient. The physicians, on average, did not see the patient until almost 11 minutes after they were roomed and ready.

EXHIBIT 4.15 Time Study 1 in Minutes

Patient	Patient Time Through Process				
	(Check-in to Ready for Doctor)	Check-in Time	Nurse Takes Chart from Window	Physician's Light On	Physician In Room
1	31	+5	+9	+6	+11
2	15	+4	+6	+4	+1
3	30	-8	+9	+6	+15
4	14	-1	+1	+10	+3
5	46	-16	+12	+9	+25
6	33	-23	+3	+13	+17
7	12	-2	+2	+5	+5
8	28	-33	+14	+9	+5
9	20	0	+5	+5	+10
10	25	-10	+15	+4	+6
11	20	-2	+1	+16	+3
12	12	-2	+5	+2	+5
13	17	+5	+1	+8	+8
14	36	-19	+4	+6	+26
15	15	+1	+13	+2	
16	15	-45	+8	+5	+2
17	35	-15	+1	+4	+30
Average	24		6.5	6.5	11

When these findings were presented to the physicians, who had initially complained about nursing staff, they realized they had to improve their own timing. Nursing staff also recognized areas of improvement. One opportunity was found in the 13-minute average time frame from check-in to the time the physician sees the patient. Once specific processes for improvement are implemented, they can be reassessed in 6 to 12 months to determine whether positive outcomes resulted.

TIME STUDY 2

A time study conducted in another practice was related to time spent on specific duties. A surgical practice wanted to look at nursing time spent in the operating room, in the office, and performing other duties. Staff included a combination of surgical technologists, RNs, and licensed practical nurses equaling five full-time-equivalent (FTE) staff. Each staff member was assigned to one physician at all times. These individuals accompanied the physician into the hospital surgical suite when he or she performed surgery (logged as operating time) and roomed patients when the physician saw patients in the office (logged as office time). Time spent on any other duty was classified as other time. Physician office time was scheduled in three to four half-day sessions per week per physician, and surgery was most often scheduled for four to five half-day sessions per week. Time sheets were used to collect the data, with the nursing staff breaking down time by hour. Individuals' time off was removed from the data tabulations. Operating room time was calculated as any time during which the nursing staff were at the hospital, rounded to the nearest hour. Assisting with office time was calculated per half day, whether time spent was a two-hour or a four-hour office visit or procedure.

The compilation of time sheets demonstrated the amount of time per 80-hour pay period that the nursing staff were in the office without office time or surgery time scheduled, documented as other duties. During other time, no nurse was dedicated exclusively to assisting the surgeon in surgery nor to assisting with an office. Each nurse was expected to put in some other duty time in the course of a normal day.

The table shown in **Exhibit 4.16** measures other duty time during a two-month time frame. (A four-month time frame was used to determine nursing staff needs.)

See, for example, total other duty time for nurse 1, which was six out of 80 hours in the first April pay period and 10.75 out of 80 hours in the second April pay period. Total nursing time spent in other duties was 90.25 out of 400 hours of the first April pay period.

Total nursing hours were calculated by multiplying hours per pay period (80) by five nursing staff, for 400 total nursing hours per pay period. Vacation time for nursing and physicians was then deducted to calculate the needed nursing hours for office and surgery. In the first pay period in April, 400 total nursing hours minus nursing vacation time (0) minus doctor out time

(8) resulted in 392 needed hours of nursing time. Total hours spent on other duty time was deducted from needed hours to obtain hours "not other" (392 − 90.25 = 301.75 for April pay period 1). This figure was then divided by 80 (an FTE for one pay period) to obtain the total staff needed for surgery and office assistance (301.75 ÷ 80 = 3.8 FTEs for April pay period 1).

EXHIBIT 4.16 Time Study 2, Other Duty Time				
	April Pay Period	April Pay Period	May Pay Period	May Pay Period
	1	2	1	2
Nurse 1	6	10.75	15.25	11
Nurse 2	23	12.75	19.75	18.75
Nurse 3	40	38.25	22.75	24
Nurse 4	7.25	12.75	9	16.75
Nurse 5	14	11	27.75	12
Total hours other time	90.25	85.5	94.5	82.5
Total nursing hours	400	400	400	400
Vacation nursing	0	(32.00)	(24.00)	(16.00)
Doctor out	(8.00)	(56.00)	(24.00)	0
Needed hours	392	312	352	384
Hours not needed	301.75	226.50	257.50	301.50
FTEs needed	3.8	2.8	3.2	3.8

Note: Pay periods are 80 hours work time.

Over the course of four months, it became obvious that nursing spent a significant amount of other time—time not spent in the operating room or office with the physician.

What do these results tell us? Nursing was either overstaffed or spending considerable amount of time in nonclinical activities (defined as non-office or non-surgery time). When the findings were presented to the physicians, they chose to continue with individual nursing staff per physician but to eliminate an office staff member, whose duties were taken over by the nursing staff.

These two time studies reveal important information about the nursing practice patterns in the two practices. Chapter 7 further explores productivity and identifies the means to determine the right amount of staff.

Chapter 5

Clinical Efficiency

Nursing plays an integral role in physician productivity and team functioning. Processes can be instituted within the nursing role that affect the physician's pace and increase efficiency. In team-based care, physicians and providers should focus on those tasks that require their skills, licensure and expertise. Because their time is the most expensive in the practice, it should be focused on seeing patients—diagnosing, performing physical exams and medical decision making. The nursing staff can complement these tasks in many ways. Efficient nursing makes the team and ultimately the whole practice more efficient, including the process of patient movement through the practice. This chapter discusses clinical efficiency as it relates to the pre-visit, visit, and post-visit phases of patient visits.

PRE-VISIT

Nursing pre-visit activities include every element of care that needs to be completed or in place when the physician enters the room to see the patient. As mentioned in Chapter 3, an efficient start to any visit is chart preparation or pre-visit planning. Other factors related to nursing efficiency in the pre-visit process include office layout, room layout, scheduling, check-in, and rooming patients, all of which are explored in this section.

Office Layout

How the office is laid out can have a huge impact on nursing productivity. Evaluating the time taken to move throughout the office to retrieve medical records and supplies, to get to and from patient rooms, and to perform other nursing tasks enables the practice to identify opportunities for optimizing office layout.

Even small steps taken to increase efficiency can go a long way toward improvement. One example is relocating nursing staff away from the front desk. Although efficiency is increased somewhat because nurses may see when patients arrive, having nurses staff the front desk is not efficient for the physician and hinders privacy when handling telephone call duty.

EXAM ROOM LAYOUT

One of the most overlooked aspects affecting nursing efficiency in a physician practice is how the examination room is laid out. For example, having all supplies within reach helps eliminate unnecessary movement, and stocking all the rooms the same way increases efficiency of both the nurse and the physician. The following questions may help in identifying exam room layout issues:

- Where is the patient in relation to the door?

- Can the nurse move around the patient without difficulty?

- Are the visitor chairs out of the way of traffic?

- Are the necessary items readily available to prepare the patient for the physician's entrance (e.g., sphygmomanometer, thermometer, stethoscope)?

- Can the supply storage doors be opened without having to move the patient and/or visitor?

- If someone enters the room during an examination, what will he or she see first—the patient's bottom during a Pap smear, perhaps?

SCHEDULING

Scheduling can have a big impact on clinical efficiency. Although nursing staff usually do not schedule office visits, they play a large part in making sure the schedule is workable. The front desk receptionist or scheduler needs guidance on scheduling concerning the following questions:

- Does the doctor have any specific instructions regarding scheduling (e.g., no pelvic exams after 3 p.m., only two procedures in one morning)?

- What patient situation requires a same-day appointment? A next-day appointment? What kind of health issue can be put off until next week?

- Should the scheduler ask specific questions of the patient? (For example, if a procedure is being scheduled, is the patient on aspirin or

Coumadin? If a yearly pelvic exam is being scheduled, when was the patient's last menstrual period?)

- Which patients can be seen by the midlevel provider rather than the physician?

- If the patient reports that he or she cannot get to the office to see the physician in a timely manner, what does the receptionist do with this patient call? (Schedule with another provider? Seek input from the nurse?)

Scheduling can be made easier for both clerical and clinical staff if clerical staff are given both guidance on and authority over the schedule. Some practices are using templates created from previous schedules to allow the scheduler to see how certain appointments were treated in the past. Use of templates provides a format for clinical staff to communicate with the schedulers on how to schedule. However, there should always be room for exceptions, and the front desk should be afforded the ability to improvise. If templates are used, it is important to look at the past three- to six-month scheduling patterns to make sure an adequate number and type of visit slots are created.

Simplifying the schedule structure also helps those who are scheduling. Some practices have 30 different visit types, and their front office staff spend more time trying to figure out what visit types to use than actually scheduling. Simplifying the scheduling process can be as easy as reducing the types of visits to less than five. Examples of simplified visit types include:

- New patient;

- Established patient;

- Established patient, new problem; and

- Procedure.

Furthermore, clarifying the characteristics of these appointment types will guide the front desk staff in determining what appointments can be scheduled with each appointment type. Schedulers can easily look at the list and know exactly how to schedule the patient.

Same-day or acute care patient visits that result from telephone calls to the office can be scheduled by receptionists if these staff are given the authority to schedule the patient instead of having to ask the nurse if the patient needs to be seen. This procedure will eliminate a phone call to the nurse and also allow the receptionist to handle the issue. A simple table prioritizing patient care needs such as acute patients (those needing to be seen today), ASAP patients (those needing appointments as soon as possible), and next-appointment patients (those needing appointments with no urgency), such as the chart shown in **Exhibit 5.1**, can be created. Allowing for same-day appointment slots on every schedule helps the front desk schedule more easily.

EXHIBIT 5.1 Scheduling Tips	
Visit Type	Symptoms or Diagnosis
Acute patient— needs to be seen today	• Uncontrolled bleeding— nosebleed, vomiting blood • Sudden severe pain • Symptoms of heart problems— chest pain, shortness of breath • Stroke symptoms— weakness on one side, slurred speech • Respiratory distress • Fever over 101.5 degrees
ASAP patient— needs to be seen as soon as possible	• Breast lump • Double vision • Flu-like symptoms for 3 days— cough with production, fever • Drainage from wound • Dizziness
Next-appointment date patient— no urgency for appointment	• Back pain • Hemorrhoids • Cold symptoms • Routine check-up

Make this chart as simple as possible and specific to your practice. The more clarity it brings, the less time nursing will spend on the phone.

Specific scheduling needs can be itemized by nursing staff to identify exactly what items of information the schedule should include so that the nursing staff know how to prepare for the patient (see **Exhibit 5.2**).

The itemized list gives clear direction to the scheduler, and the examples show exactly what nursing is asking to be included in the schedule. Once again, do not make the list so complicated that it will be impossible to follow.

EXHIBIT 5.2 Visit Type Explanation		
	What Should Be Included in Scheduling Notes	Example
New patients	• Reason for visit • Referring doctor (if specialist • Any testing or films (where taken) • Other pertinent information	Specialist Abn mammo, Dr. Jones, mammo 2/07 at Green Hospital, pt told location and to bring films Primary care Cough for two weeks w/ production, CXR at urgent care; pt concerned about CA
Established patients	• Reason for visit • Referring doctor (if specialist) • Past procedure or surgery and date, if applicable • Testing	Specialist Postop, chole 2/1, Green Hospital, Dr. Jones Primary care follow-up hypertension, lytes 3/1

Scheduling preferences of physicians can be accommodated easily by creating a cheat sheet, such as that shown in **Exhibit 5.3**, detailing each physician's specific requests. Using this sheet, staff will know exactly what they may and may not do regarding scheduling.

Much of the information related to scheduling procedures may be known only by the scheduler, and when that person leaves the practice suddenly the "known" information is lost. Documenting these preferences allows everyone in the practice who needs them to have access to them.

The simpler the schedule, the more likely it will work efficiently. Regular discussions between nursing and schedulers are very helpful. If scheduling issues arise, discuss them among clinical and scheduling staff, determine what triggered them, and change the process if necessary and try again.

Another option in scheduling is open access, which can be a schedule left completely open, pre-filled with chronic disease patients only or have a certain percentage of pre-filled slots. Patients are then given more access when they call in for today's needs. Regardless of the scheduling option used, communication between the nursing staff and schedulers is vital.

EXHIBIT 5.3 Schedule Preferences

	Doctor 1	Doctor 2	Doctor 3	Doctor 4
Pelvic/Pap	2-3/day	2-3/day	1-2/day	2-3/day
Procedures lesion removal	3-4/week, prefers 9 a.m.	3-4/week	3, Tuesdays only	1-2/day
Treadmill	1/week	1/week- Tuesdays	2/week- 1st appt in afternoon	None
OB patients	2/day	3/day	4/day	1/day
Add-on acute patients	6/day	3/day, at end of office	4/day, 1- 1:30 p.m.	8/day
Complete physicals	1/day	4, Wednesday, a.m.	3, Thursday, p.m.	1-2/day

CHART PREPARATION

Chart preparation (chart prep) can be as simple as having the chart, either electronic or paper, ready at the time of the visit, or it can be as detailed as reviewing the chart and gathering multiple pieces of information prior to the visit. Physicians should be consulted about their requirements for chart prep regarding specific patients. An example of chart prep for a surgical or an oncology practice is shown in **Exhibit 5.4**. Pre-visit planning can be performed by nursing prior to the visit. It allows nursing staff to review the last visit; gather any tests performed since the last visit; or alert the patient to bring X-ray films, medications, or other items to the appointment. A more efficient and cost-effective approach might be to designate one person to do the initial review of records, make sure all the necessary information is on the record, and request those items that are not in place prior to the visit. This person should have a good understanding of diagnoses and testing and be able to think clinically about what may be needed for the visit.

Chart prep may be simplified if the physician follows a certain routine. A specialist in one practice always dictates a letter to the referring physician after the visit listing all tests and procedures he has performed for that patient. That letter allows the chart prep person to easily update the chart. In another practice, chart prep is aided by a note created by the physician itemizing steps needed before the next visit. The example shown in **Exhibit 5.5** is from an oncology practice that uses a flow sheet for each visit. The sheet is designed to make clear the tests needed for the next visit.

EXHIBIT 5.4 Chart Preparation per Diagnosis		
	Questions to Ask Patient and/or Referral (Dates and Where Done)	Chart Preparation— Needed Prior to Appointment
Abdominal mass; 1st visit to general surgeon	• EGD • Abdominal sonogram • CT scan • Referring doc and PCP if different • Colonoscopy Have patient bring CT films	• EGD and biopsy results • Sonogram reports • CT scan film and reports • Lab results • Colonoscopy report • Consult report
Breast cancer; 1st visit to oncologist	• Past mamograms or breast sonograms • Biopsy, when and where • Surgery, when and where • Recent lab	• Radiology reports for mammogram and sonogram • Operative reports • Path reports • Consult reports from surgeons • Most recent lab if done

Note: CT= computed tomography; EGD = esophagogastroduodenoscopy; path = pathology; PCP=primary care physician

Processes should be established so that the appropriate test results are documented on the chart prior to the follow-up appointment. How the test result moves through the practice is important to understand. Are all test results faxed to a certain fax machine at the practice, are they sent electronically through the EMR, do all arrive by mail, or is a combination of methods used? Are the results on the physician's inbox or desk awaiting signature? Are they held in a file awaiting the next visit? Are they filed immediately? Are they with the chart? All of these variables should be known and then explored to determine the most efficient means of routing and chart prep completion.

EXHIBIT 5.5 Oncology Visit Note

Date_____	Return Appt	Transfusion ____ units
Name_____	Dr_____	___platelets ___Packed RBCS
Dx_____	PA_____	Other _____
ICD_____		

Chemo and IV fluids:

_____

_____

change to:

_____

_____

☐ IV fluids:

_____

☐ IV antibiotics:

_____

☐ Other:

_____

_____

Injection orders:

☐ Neupogen _____mcg

Continue same orders

150 - 300 - 480 - 600

Daily - M - T - W - Th - F - Sat - Sun

Other_____

☐ Epogen _____ units

Continue same orders

10,000 - 20,000 - 30,000 - 40,000

Daily - M - T - W - Th - F - Sat - Sun

Other_____

☐ Fragmin 5,000 Udaily x _____ days

☐ Other

Lab	Today	Next Visit	Weekly	Other	Radiology Test	Order (when, special, etc).
CBC					CT head	
Chem prof					CT chest	
LDH					CT abd	
PT					Bone Scan	
CEA					MRI brain	
CA 125					MRI thoracic	
TSH					Xray chest	
PSA					Mammogram	
UA						

RX:	Other Tests:
	Consult other doctors:
Samples:	
Teaching needed:	Other:
Consult: dietitian social worker	Dr Signature _____

CHECK-IN

The next step in the pre-visit process is patient check-in. Check-in involves duties performed by the clerical staff, including greeting the patient, collecting the copayment, and notifying nursing of the patient's arrival.

The greatest variability from practice to practice may occur in the notification step. Every practice has a different method of notifying nursing, which may be one of the following:

- The receptionist alerts the nursing staff by phone.

- The receptionist places or takes the chart to a designated area.

- The charge ticket is printed in the nursing area.

- The nursing staff are alerted through the electronic medical record (EMR) or practice management system.

- The receptionist turns on a designated light that alerts the nursing staff.

- To determine whether the method chosen is the most efficient for your practice, ask the following questions:

- Are any wasteful steps performed?

- Does someone often wait on someone else?

- Is the process timely?

Efficient check-in allows enough time to gather all the pertinent information from the patient as well as quick and seamless movement of the patient to the nursing staff. It should resemble the flowchart shown in **Exhibit 5.6**.

Late arrivals or no-show patients can slow down the check-in process. Patients who show up on the wrong day or at the wrong time and those who walk in for treatment without an appointment also affect check-in timing. Having a procedure in place that directs staff on how to handle these patients can reduce the confusion at the front desk and can allow the patients to be treated in a matter-of-fact, routine manner. One approach to documenting these patient visits is shown in **Exhibit 5.7**.

EXHIBIT 5.6 Efficient Check-In

Patient arrives at practice. Front desk processes patient

Charge ticket placed on chart and taken to nursing

Charge ticket printed in nursing area, placed on chart by nursing

Patient called back to exam room by nursing

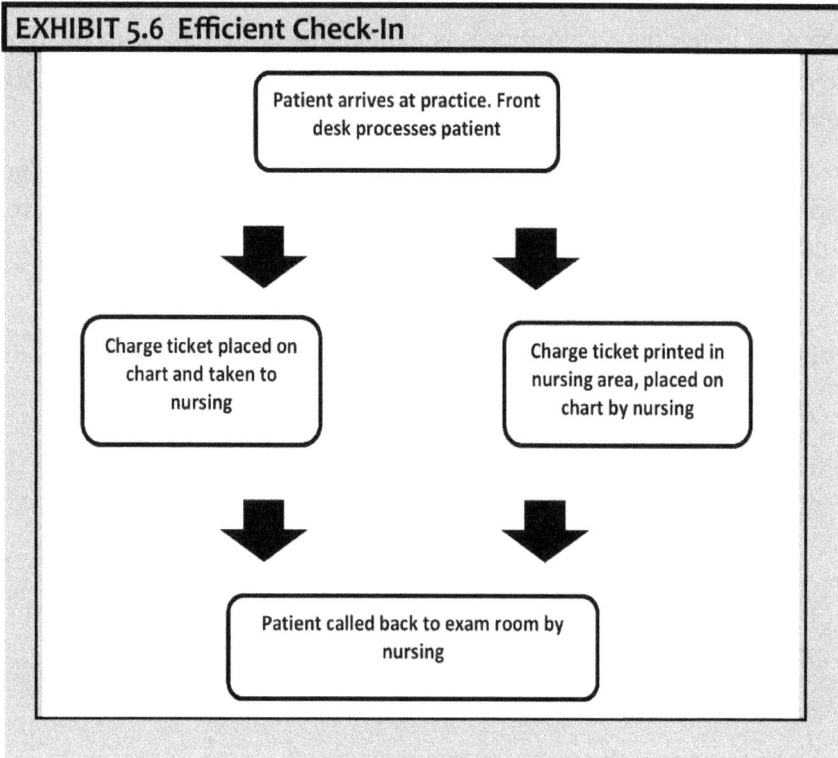

ROOMING PATIENTS

Following check-in, nursing places the patient in an examination room and performs duties required prior to the physician's entrance into the room. This component of the pre-visit stage includes a number of steps that should be performed quickly but thoroughly. By evaluating each step in the process, opportunities for improvement may be noted. In one practice, it was found that nurses spent several minutes helping elderly patients on and off the weight scale. The simple suggestion was made to lower the scale to be flush with the floor so that older patients could more easily use it, saving a significant amount of time.

EXHIBIT 5.7 No-Show and Late-Arriving Patients

Patients who have a scheduled appointment may fail to show up or arrive late for that appointment. The following procedure will be used to document those patients.

No-show patients:

1. A patient is a no-show patient if he or she does not arrive for the appointment 15 minutes past the appointment time.

2. Each patient is researched to ensure the patient is not in the hospital.

3. If the patient is identified as a no-show patient, a no-show is marked in the practice management system.

4. The nursing staff are notified, and they attempt to contact the patient to reschedule.

5. The physician is notified of the no-show patient if the patient cannot be reached.

6. Patients are allowed two no-show visits before being considered for termination from the practice.

Late-arriving patients:

1. A patient is considered a no-show patient if he or she does not show for the appointment 15 minutes past the appointment time (see the procedure for no-show patients above.)

2. If the patient arrives for the appointment more than 15 minutes past the appointment time, the physician is notified and makes a decision as to whether he or she will see this patient.

3. if the physician chooses not to see the patient, the patient is rescheduled.

A checklist may be used to streamline the rooming process for nursing staff. In one family practice, a checklist form was used to ensure that all pertinent information was gathered. The use of the form also increased the physician's efficiency in dictation—she no longer had to search through the chart—and it   enhanced communication flow between nursing and the physician during pre- and post-visit activities. This can be done in an electronic format also. (See **Exhibit 5.8**.)

EXHIBIT 5.8 Pre-visit Sheet

Pre-visit Sheet

Name_____ DOB_____Date_____

Nursing: reason for visit_____

_____

T_____P_____R_____BP_____sitting BP_____standing_____

Ht_____Wt_____ Pharmacy_____

Allergies: NKDA_____
Injury: Y N _____Work comp: Y N

Medication check: Y N _____Immunization check: Y N

Physician orders:

Lab: CBC CMP BMP UA Strep Hbg A1C T4 PSA Lipid

X-ray:_____ Referral:_____

Procedure: _____

Return appt: _____ Samples:_____

Rx:_____

Many practices have the front office and nursing staff fill out part of the medical record by collecting certain information, such as social, medical or surgical history, chronic disease or preventive care milestones, and to discuss advance directives with patients. Filling out a checklist, either electronically or in paper form, that includes these items is a good place to start this process and an easy reminder to staff rooming patients.

For the step of alerting the physician that the patient is ready to be seen, the use of flags or lights can be helpful. In several practices, a light is turned on when the patient is ready for the physician. In other practices, flags attached to the various rooms indicate where the patient is in the process (e.g., roomed and ready for the physician, lab needed, nursing follow-up needed), streamlining communication. Notifying the physician through the EMR is also used.

Anticipating the physician's needs can assist with patient flow. If the patient will need lab work, a radiology visit, or prescriptions, referrals and prepared refill requests can be placed ready for the physician to access. The presence of pre-scriptions—electronic or paper—can be included on a nursing checklist.

EVIDENCE-BASED GUIDELINES

For many prevalent diseases, there is growing research related to standardiz-ing the treatment of those conditions. These are in the form of evidence-based guidelines for diseases such as diabetes, hypertension, depression, ADHD, etc. Often times, nursing staff can carry out the evidence-based guidelines through the use of standing orders. For instance, an evidence based guideline for diabetes is that every stable diabetic will have an Hgb A1c blood test yearly. A standing order could be written related to that guideline. The nursing staff can use the standing order to complete the test prior to the patient seeing the physician if the patient has a diagnosis of diabetes and has not had a test in the past year.

Standing orders can also be used for preventive care such as mammograms or-dered for all females yearly over the age of 50 or childhood immunizations per evidence based guideline adopted by the physicians.

VISIT

Nursing visit activities include those pertaining to the patient while the patient is still present in the office. These activities take place in the areas of medication administration, nursing procedures, supplies, and patient education.
Medication Administration

A medication record completed for each patient's chart is a helpful tool in man-aging medication administration. A good medication record clearly identifies a patient's current medications and changes made during the course of treatment. Primary care offices may benefit from a more detailed listing, such as that shown in **Exhibit 5.9**, considering they typically treat the patient over several years.

This example provides a straightforward list of medications the patient is taking or has taken at any given time. Many EMRs have similar medication records.

EXHIBIT 5.9 Medication List

Name: _____

DOB: _____

Allergies: Penicillin _____

_____

_____

_____

_____

Review of Medications

Medication	Dosage	1/07/06	2/21/07	5/22/07	11/26/07	4/15/08	10/02/08
Allegra 60 mg	1 tab bid	X	X	X	X		
Allegra 60 mg	1 tab q d					X	X
Sudafed 30 mg	1 tab in a.m.		X	X	X	X	X
Nasonex spray	2 sprays daily each nostril			X	X	X	
Lasix 20 mg	1 tab q a.m.	X	X	X			
Vit B-12 Injection	1 x/month-mid-month	X	X			X	X

It is advised to avoid marking out or removing medications from the patient's medication list that are no longer used; this past history is often helpful in treating current and future health issues. With every visit, the nursing staff should ask about any changes in the patient's medications. It may be difficult for the patient to remember medication names and dosages, so having the patient bring his or her medications to the appointment may ensure accuracy in this step. Some physicians ask nursing to obtain a complete medication listing, while other physicians personally review medications with the patient. In addition to prescription drugs, sample, over-the-counter, and supplement medications should be listed on the medication sheet. The front office can also streamline this process by printing out a medication listing for each patient to review and be ready to answer the questions about medications.

When a patient's medication changes, either during the office visit or as a result of telephone triage, his or her medication log should be updated. Patient medication logs are often used during subsequent phone triage, office visits, and admission to the hospital setting. Keeping an updated medication log is more efficient than leafing through 10 pages of progress notes to find all the medications in the patient's treatment history. The physician's assistance with log updates helps ensure the medication record is complete. And, of course, keeping patient records in an electronic format saves time.

Efficiency in medication administration is driven by the type of medication-related supplies and the location of those supplies. Medication administration cannot be hurried, but it can be made more efficient if the necessary supplies are readily available and user friendly. Location of the supplies should be in close proximity to the site where the supplies will be used. It is not efficient for nursing staff or physicians to walk clear across the clinic to obtain samples or a medication for an injection. When determining a location for medication supplies, keep in mind that medications should be kept out of reach of patients; medication storage in exam rooms should be limited. Supplies that require much effort to use should also be reduced or eliminated. One nurse simply could not work with a metal tubex for injections despite thorough teaching and practice. She had always used a plastic tubex and preferred it over the metal. The practice purchased a plastic tubex, and this simple act gave her a tool that improved her efficiency.

When considering patient flow and timing related to medication administration, bear in mind that patients should be kept in the office after an injection for an adequate amount of time to ensure that they have no reaction to the medications. This time frame varies by medication, the frequency of injections, and the patient's history of taking the medication or past side effects. The patient can be asked to wait in the reception area for the time period with instructions to notify nursing when he or she is leaving or if symptoms occur.

NURSING PROCEDURES

Most nursing procedures, such as dressing changes, suture removal, casting, or catheter irrigation, are carried out in the exam room after the patient has been seen by the physician. The main consideration in performing procedures efficiently is how the room is stocked. The room should be stocked with adequate supplies for those procedures that occur frequently. However, avoid overstocking. It makes no sense to stock a room with casting material if castings are rare, for example. Due to the cost and volume of casting supplies, a separate room should actually be set up for this procedure. In short, when stocking exam rooms, think about all the nursing procedures that will be performed in the room and then stock the room accordingly.

SUPPLIES

Stocking rooms on a regular basis for those periods when the physician is seeing patients in the office saves valuable time. Maintaining a regular stocking schedule helps identify when to stock the rooms, and a list of items posted in each cabinet reveals what is needed. Do not assume that all clinical staff know what and when to stock—they do not.

In offices where physicians move among different exam rooms, create a common stocking area from room to room: a particular drawer, a designated tub on top of a counter, a specific cabinet, and so forth. Using the same stocking approach and making exam room supply areas similar help avoid confusion as to where items are located.

PATIENT EDUCATION

Many efforts can be taken to make patient education tools more efficient, starting with the location of these tools. For an orthopedic office in which total knee replacement, total hip replacement, or arthroscopy are the main surgical procedures performed, patient information handouts related to these procedures can be kept in the exam room for distribution during the appointment. For a general surgeon who performs at least a dozen different procedures, on the other hand, keeping the various relevant handouts in the exam room is not efficient. However, the location of these education tools should still be within easy reach of the exam room.

A cost-effective measure may be to develop education materials that are unique to the practice if certain procedures are performed frequently. If all the physicians perform hernia repairs and they are in agreement about the patient instructions, the office can prepare a nicely printed sheet or booklet to give to patients. In addition to helping save costs, this approach enhances the accuracy and effectiveness of patient education because it is tailored to the particular office.

Several Internet sites provide a great amount of information about procedures and surgeries. Patients can be directed to the practice's website, if the practice is operating one, with links to preferred external websites, or they can be provided a neatly printed handout to take home listing those websites. Preprinted handouts can be made available for those patients who do not have Internet access, but you may find that a large percentage of patients will want to do some exploring of their health issue on their own.

Even if you have prepared patient education tools, nursing staff still must take time to briefly explain the reading material. Make sure both nursing and telephone triage staff read and understand what they are teaching. In addition, ensure the accuracy of the handouts. Phone call volume will increase if handouts are not correct or explained fully.

Making sure the patient understands how to manage their disease or condition between office visits is also key in patient education. Do they know how to use the glucometer and record the readings? Do they know which exercise activities they can follow? Are there any foods they should avoid or actions they should take to mitigate problems? Do they know what symptoms indicate they are having problems, such as a congestive heart failure patient needing to weigh daily and seeing a two-pound weight gain? Simple handouts can be created for chronic disease patients that touch on diet, exercise and monitoring between visits.

POST-VISIT

Post-visit nursing activities most often are performed after the patient leaves the office but, depending on the situation, may be performed during the visit. These activities involve many areas of the practice, including handling telephone duty and triage, physician orders, community resources, referrals, diagnostic testing and follow-up, procedure and surgery scheduling, prescription drug program information, Family Medical Leave Act (FMLA) or other paperwork, pharmaceutical representative visits, quality-of-care standards, patient satisfaction, and clinical trials.

TELEPHONE MANAGEMENT

Every practice uses a different method for managing nursing phone calls. Various ways to handle these calls include the following:

- All phone calls go to voice mail and are picked up later.
- Clinical staff answer the phone call, review the chart, and call the patient back.
- The nurse fields the phone call as he or she looks up the patient and accompanying notes in the EMR.

The last option is probably the most effective and time efficient.

To improve nursing staff efficiency, for all phone calls taken, a note regarding the call should be attached to the record and the record sent to the nurse. To improve efficiency for the office staff, the phone call should be answered by the nurse, who looks at the record.. Nursing should be wary of fielding phone calls without having access to the medical record if for no other reason than to document the call.

If a phone triage nurse is used, a phone call should be directed to the nursing staff after it is screened by the front office. If the nurse is taking care of only one doctor's calls, having the medical record available is important, but the one-to-one relationship will likely enable the nurse to identify and answer the patient's questions and document the call later.

In one practice, instead of having one person responsible for phone calls for that physician, anyone taking the phone call was responsible for asking the physician how to proceed. This method created chaos. To ease the situation, this practice could assign a phone triage position and/or a primary nurse/assistant should be assigned to be the gatekeeper for any phone calls. All messages are routed to him or her, and that individual asks the physician about all of them in one session.

Another problem identified in a practice was that people frequently gave out the back-line phone number to patients and outside agencies. This disclosure creates an opportunity for outside agencies to gain inappropriate access. It became a problem for one practice when a nurse was out sick for an extended period of time. He had given out his back-line number, and consequently, all of his contacts called that number instead of the main line, creating a delay in getting the call answered. A clear policy on using and disclosing information about the back line should be created.

PHONE TRIAGE

Nursing phone triage is the process in which the nurse, after discussing the patient's health situation with the patient, makes a determination as to the treatment protocol. This may involve one or more of the following activities:

- Symptom assessment
- Counseling
- Home treatment advice
- Referral information provision
- Disease management
- Crisis intervention
- Physician referral management
- Health information provision
- Appointment scheduling
- Authorization service

To provide effective nursing phone triage, the nurse should have:

- excellent communication skills;
- critical thinking skills;
- the ability to handle stressful situations;
- the capacity to function independently;
- varied clinical experience, including hospital; and
- the ability to document conversations and conduct patient teaching.

Phone triage requires the use of the nursing process: assessment, diagnosis, treatment, and evaluation. Here it is important to distinguish between nursing diagnosis and medical diagnosis. Nursing diagnosis involves the nurse assessing the patient, gathering both subjective and objective information, and using clinical decision making to form a decision about next steps. One example is the patient who calls to report symptoms (objective data) and how he or she feels (subjective data). Based on both types of information, the nurse determines whether the patient needs to be seen by a physician or can self-manage their symptoms with clinical advice.

In contrast, medical diagnosis occurs when the physician takes an after-hours call from a patient reporting symptoms. The physician diagnoses the disease and prescribes medications over the phone as necessary.

True nursing phone triage carries the risk of liability. Consider this example of a mother who calls to report her infant is crying constantly because, she thinks, the baby is not getting enough breast milk. The nurse advises the mother to start the child on rice cereal to supplement the breast milk. Two days later, the infant is brought to the local hospital's emergency department and diagnosed with meningitis, a serious condition that can lead to death. The nurse and practice in this case may be considered liable for the misdiagnosis and delay in treatment.

To reduce the liability risk, whether and how to conduct nursing phone triage should be carefully considered. Well-designed procedures, staff competency verification, and documentation guidelines should be in place prior to implementation. Phone triage–related liability may be reduced by implementing procedures that address the following areas:

- Risk management (handling the health issues of minors, angry callers, noncompliance, power failure backup systems, issues concerning nursing across state lines, etc.)

- Process management (defining guidelines; fielding calls that do not fit into a defined guideline; handling medications, lab testing, and emergency calls; prioritizing calls, making referrals, etc.)

- Clinic issues management (determining who receives the call, who accesses the records, when the patient is seen, etc.)

- Numerous resources are available for developing guidelines, and guidelines can also be created wholly in-house. Either way, these guidelines should be evidence based and follow nationally recognized standards of care. They can be either symptom or disease based. An example of a guideline for heartburn is shown in **Exhibit 5.10**.

EXHIBIT 5.10 Phone Triage Guideline

Heartburn

Assessment:	Plan
• Heartburn 1 hour after eating a heavy or spicy meal. • Pain intense, lasts for a few hours • Patient taking antacids	• Avoid foods that are spicy, acidic, tomato based, or fatty • Avoid tea, cola, caffeine • Eat moderate amounts of food without overfilling • Eliminate tobacco • Do not exercise after eating • Do not lie down for 3–4 hours after eating • Avoid wearing tight belts • Schedule an appointment if these measures do not work

Staff competency is vital to making phone triage successful. The most important competency is licensure. Only registered nurses or experienced licensed practical nurses should attempt phone triage. Phone triage requires critical thinking skills and a background in the nursing process. Experienced nurses make better decisions than new graduates because they have been exposed during their career to a number of different situations. A continuous monitoring system should be implemented and a review by a supervising physician of all phone calls should be conducted to determine the abilities and knowledge base of the triage nurse.

PHYSICIAN ORDERS

It is important to establish a procedure for handling physician orders in the practice. Too often, it is assumed that physicians have discussed parameters with nursing staff only to discover later that the nurse gave an unauthorized order to a patient.

The physician order procedure should address the following questions:

- Who can give orders (nurses only, unlicensed personnel, physicians only)?

- How are orders transmitted (verbally, faxed, e-mailed, mailed)?

- Are any standing orders in place? When can they be used, and who can use them?

- How are prescriptions renewed (through a pharmacy; by the patient; via fax, phone, or by electronic methods)?

- Can the nursing staff renew certain medications?

- Can the nursing staff use the physician's signature stamp for certain orders?

- Can the nursing staff initiate certain treatments?

- Can the nursing staff give out medication samples if the patient asks for them?

- How recently must the patient have been seen to have a medication refilled (within three months, within one year)?

For many practices, the most frequent physician order given is for refills. In some practices, each physician uses a different method to refill medications. Although it takes some effort, the physicians and nursing staff can reach agreement on how the refill process should be handled. A procedure to establish the ground rules for refills can include the following guidelines:

- The dosage of the medication must match the medication log, the physician's dictation, or a message contained in the chart.

- The patient must still under the physician's care and not dismissed from the practice.

- All patients must have been seen within the last 12 months.

- If the patient has not been seen within the indicated time, a month's prescription will be given and the patient is required to make an appointment.

- Generic medications are approved unless otherwise stated by the physician. Certain drugs are listed that cannot be refilled in generic form.

- Any medication not listed on the refill table (see **Exhibit 5.11**) has to be approved by the physician.

- The procedure and refill table are reviewed by the physicians yearly.

- One-year prescription refills can only be given by the physician.

- Narcotic prescription refills can only be given by the physician.

A refill table, such as that shown in **Exhibit 5.11**, can establish guidelines per medication classification for how often the patient needs to be seen in the office, how often lab work needs to be done, and how many refills can be given.

In other practices, the physician may want to see every prescription refill request or designate a midlevel provider to handle refill requests. If a midlevel provider is on staff, a protocol should be established to avoid misunderstandings between the provider and the physician. Refills requests and refill orders should be documented in the medical record.

A primary care practice can become inundated with patient phone calls related to refill requests. One helpful option to manage them is to only take refill requests from the pharmacy; the patient is told to call the pharmacy to trigger the request. If a fax machine is used to receive pharmacy refill requests, it should be located by the medical records area so that the appropriate record can be pulled to place with the refill. Electronic handling of refills is easier for the provider to manage than are paper-based refills.

EXHIBIT 5.11 Medication Refills and Orders

	Physician Visit Frequency	Lab Order Frequency	Refills
Hypo-thyriodism	Every 12 months	☐ TSH yearly if stable ☐ Dosage change - consult provider	Enough to last until required follow-up
Hyper-lipidemia	Every 12 months	☐ Lipid profile and ALT/AST 2 months after starting or increasing dose, and then every 3 months X 2, then every 6 months X 1, then every 12 months ☐ Medicare - see Medicare lipid coverage ☐ Niacin - liver function tests annually	☐ If LDL< 130 w/ no risk factors - refill enough to last until next follow up ☐ If LDL< 100 and if cardiac disease or diabetes - refill enough to last until next follow-up
Hormone replacement	☐ Well woman visit once a year ☐ Current on mammogram		Give enough to last until next exam
Contraception	☐ Yearly exam with Pap ☐ Current on mammogram		Up to 12 months to last until next required exam
Coumadin	☐ Every 6 months ☐ Dosage changes as per Dr.	☐ INR every month ☐ INR in therapeutic range	☐ Enough until next appointment (6 months max)
Allergy injections	☐ Order from allergist ☐ Patient at this clinic	Medication and orders from allergist	
Flu vaccine	☐ 6 months or older ☐ At risk ☐ Pregnant women past the 3rd month of pregnancy	☐ 6 months-8 years: 2 doses one month apart for 1st immunization ☐ <35 months: 0.25 ml IM ☐ >3 years: 0.5 ml IM	☐ No egg allergies ☐ No past reactions

Another way to reduce phone calls for refills is to ask the patient during the appointment about refills. If a pre-visit checklist is used to check in the patient, the nurse rooming the patient can be prompted to ask about refills. A final option is to have a refill tablet or sign placed in the exam room that alerts the patient to ask for refills. If a tablet is used, the patient can tear off the sheet after writing down those refills he or she needs (see **Exhibit 5.12**).

EXHIBIT 5.12 Refill Sheet

Refills needed:

Please list medications in need of refill.

Other physician order issues include giving verbal orders and using physician signature stamps. Ordering treatment verbally should be limited by requiring the nursing staff to fax any orders with the physician's signature. This procedure helps avoid misunderstandings and reduces exposure to liability.

A physician's signature stamp is commonly used on orders in a physician's office. Because such a stamp may be accessible to any number of people in the office, a procedure should be implemented and the physician's approval for its use obtained before nursing staff can use it. The procedure may indicate, for example, that a stamp can be used for orders for lab work and radiology, for referrals to outside agencies or to outside health care providers (home health, durable medical equipment, etc.), or for claim filing. The physician should formalize the specific parameters for use of the stamp with a document such as that shown in **Exhibit 5.13**.

As indicated in the sample authorization displayed in **Exhibit 5.13**, it is always a good idea for the person who uses the stamp to initial next to the stamped physician's signature as authentication of the stamp. Bear in mind that some regulations require the original physician's signature.

Some nursing staff can initiate treatment without obtaining consent from a physician because they have gained expertise from extensive training and experience on the job. For example, when a patient calls in with a cough that has been persistent for several weeks, the nurse, based on his or her experience working with the physician for many years, knows that the physician will want to view a chest X-ray of the patient before seeing the patient in the office. The nurse orders a chest X-ray without first obtaining the physician's consent. The nurse initiating treatment saves the physician time, but remember that when the nurse orders that chest X-ray, he or she is actually practicing medicine without a written order. To avoid potential misunderstandings, patient safety breaches, and liability risks, a list of protocols should be in place that the nursing staff can follow. Such a list also allows other staff to work with a physician in the absence of his or her nurse.

EXHIBIT 5.13 Authorization to Use Stamp

I, _____, authorize the use of my signature stamp by my assigned nurse _____.
This stamp may be used for the following purposes under my general supervision:

- Physician orders for laboratory or radiology
- Referrals to outside health care providers
- Orders to outside health care providers

The nurse will initial the stamped signature to authenticate the order.

_____   _____
Physician signature   Date

COMMUNITY RESOURCES

The community resources discussed in this context are external health care providers, specialists, therapists, vendors, and others to whom the patient is referred for specific types of treatment or care.

Each physician will most likely have preferences in using certain community resources (e.g., which home health agency, which specialist, which physical therapist). Having a cheat sheet readily available to nursing staff that includes a list of all approved community resources and their main contact name and phone number speeds up the process of contacting these organizations.

Coding for reimbursement is an important issue when referring patients to community resources (e.g., lab, therapy). Make sure your nursing staff meet on a regular basis with a coder. The coder can create a simple sheet listing the most frequently used codes and serve as a resource for nursing in the community resource coding process.

In a family practice, a separate position may be needed to facilitate coordination of community resources. The individual fulfilling those duties can be located in an office next to the check-out area for patients' convenience.

REFERRAL MANAGEMENT AND TRACKING

Referrals to physicians or agencies require management by the nursing staff. When the referral is initially made, the nursing staff communicate to the referral physician the reason the patient is referred. This communication usually involves the nursing staff faxing or sending medical records of any pertinent clinical findings to the new physician or agency. For a patient referred to a home health agency for treatment of a wound, for example, the nursing staff must identify the wound location, treatment plans, and follow-up care needed. To help ensure better patient care, the nurse can fax a medication listing, a note detailing latest progress, and the physician's order to the agency.

Nursing responsibility related to community resources does not end with completing the referral. Making sure that the patient is seen by the referral entity in a timely manner and that the physician's orders are carried out are also part of the nurse's duties. Consulting physicians usually report back to the referring physician, and these reports must be tracked. Home health agencies send a plan of care to the physician for signature. To aid in monitoring the care plans of those patients referred to outside agencies or to other physicians, a tracking log or electronic report can be used.

Why is this monitoring important or necessary? Say the patient is told by the physician that he is being referred to a surgeon to discuss a mass in his abdomen. The referring physician has a strong suspicion that the patient has metastatic disease. However, the patient is never called by the surgeon and therefore assumes that some kind of mistake has been made in the diagnosis. Unless that referral is tracked, assurance that the patient is properly treated cannot be obtained. Finally, never assume the patient will follow or understand the instructions given.

Likewise, the consulting or referral physician carries responsibility for the patient's treatment process. If the patient is unable to be scheduled, the consulting physician has a responsibility to inform the referring physician of the situation. The following example shows the importance of a referral physician accepting this responsibility: A surgeon is faxed a referral for a breast cancer patient from a primary care physician. After repeated attempts to contact the patient, the surgeon calls the primary care physician to inform her of his inability to schedule the patient. The primary care office is aware of circumstances that made the patient unreachable at that time (she was out of town attending the funeral of a loved one) and is able to put the surgeon in contact with the patient.

For those patients who self-refer to another physician, tracking of encounters with the new physician can be helpful in understanding the true picture of the patient's health. Asking patients to forward a report to your office is usually all that is needed, as patients typically want their physician to know what is happening to them regarding their health situation.

DIAGNOSTIC TESTING

With all the different insurance company requirements regarding use of particular diagnostic service companies, diagnostic testing can be a disaster waiting to happen. Nurses need to know a phenomenal amount of information related to reimbursement and to keep up to date with insurance company rules, such as which insurance company will allow which lab to perform diagnostic work. Attempt to work with a lab that takes all insurance (essentially a perfect-world scenario). If such a lab does not exist in your area, create a list of labs that the insurance companies require, such as that shown in **Exhibit 5.14**. Also, ask the manager of the testing site if either faxing or electronically sending the order is an option.

EXHIBIT 5.14 Required Lab Protocol by Insurance Company

Insurance Company	Required Lab
Aetna	1 Lab
Blue Cross	Check on card
BlueAdvantage	2 Lab
Blue Care	2 Lab
Cigna	3 Lab
Coventry	1 Lab
Principal	Check on card

Another problem with coordinating diagnostic testing is the need to give the testing center a diagnosis with the ordered tests. A cheat sheet can be created to assist the nurse in the major diagnoses that he or she frequently uses when ordering tests. In addition, precertification from the insurance company may be needed for certain radiology tests. Obtaining assistance from the testing center to gain precertification often results in timely action. The center wants your business and will help you in the referral process.

FOLLOW-UP ON DIAGNOSTIC TESTING

If a diagnostic test is ordered, the results should be documented to ensure they are received. Any liability carrier will agree that great risk is involved in not following up on tests ordered. It takes commitment by the nursing staff to ensure testing is complete and the results received. Follow-up can be done in numerous ways, including the following:

- The nurse keeps a copy of the lab order until the test result is received.

- An electronic or paper tracking log is kept by the nurse, or nursing staff, who documents the date results were received. This method works well if all test results come into one location at the physician practice office—through a fax machine, through the EMR, or fax server or by mail.

- Some physicians might think their memory is good enough to mentally keep track of all the tests they order and whether they have seen the results of each. Many people overestimate their capacity to remember, and it only takes one missed chest X-ray showing a spot on a lung to generate a lawsuit. Therefore, it is advised to keep a diagnostic test tracking log, such as the one shown in **Exhibit 5.15**. This log clearly reveals any missing test results. (The same log may also be used for referral tracking.)

Nursing staff may have to track tests that are ordered yearly (mammograms, colonoscopies, etc.). Most electronic systems have the capability to track annual testing and to generate a reminder letter, text or portal message for the patient. Keeping a small card file works well for an individual physician setting up a paper tracking system.

Although patients are expected to be a partner in their medical regime, it still falls to the physician and staff to ensure testing is done appropriately and follow-up is provided.

EXHIBIT 5.15 Diagnostic Test Tracking Log

Date	Patient Name	DOB	Test Ordered	Test Received	Disposition
5/22/08	Patient 1	10/22/66	CBC	5/23/08	Given to doctor with chart
5/22/08	Patient 2	3/14/22	CT abd	5/26/08	Called pt for appt 5/27
5/22/08	Patient 3	4/15/45	CT chest	5/27/08	Talked to doctor, more tests ordered, call to patient
6/25/08	Patient 25	6/26/38	Bone scan		
6/25/08	Patient 26	2/28/62	CBC	6/26/08	Given to doctor with chart
6/25/08	Patient 27	4/14/22	MRI head		

Follow-up from Hospitalizations / Care Transitions

In order to assist patients with a smooth transition home after a hospitalization, emergency room visit and/or a nursing home stay, the nursing staff can make a phone call to selected patients. A list of patients with their diagnosis dismissed from the hospital on a daily basis is the first step. Nursing can call each of those patients, especially chronic care patients, to ensure they have a follow-up appointment, know what medications to take and self-care instructions. Self-care would include any monitoring or actions the patient needs to take to ensure they won't be re-hospitalized, including what signs would indicate they are having problems.

CARE MANAGEMENT

If a patient needs additional support, the care manager may work with the patient between visits to help them better understand and monitor their illness. This could include regular phone calls, home visits and/or office visits dependent upon the needs of the patient. Patient education is a big part of these visits as well as clinical decision making. Usually RNs are asked to take on this role if the patient is at high risk for hospitalization or exacerbation. A care plan is used often to make the care more efficient and focused. This can be documented in the medical record for all to see. The care manager can be more efficient and effective if she/he is included in huddles or office visits that pertain to the patient. Integration of the care manager role requires discussion prior to and during activities.

SCHEDULING PROCEDURES OR SURGERIES

Many procedures or surgeries require insurance precertification, depending on where the procedure is performed. Precertification is a very important element of the practice for the billing office, but it does not carry the same importance for nursing staff. For that reason, if possible, the task of seeking precertification should be placed with the billing office. A hand-off sheet can be created to assist in ensuring the billing office has all the information needed.

If a physician performs surgery or procedures in more than one location, scheduling can be a challenge. The use of block time for one physician or a group of physicians makes scheduling for multiple locations efficient if volume of procedures or surgeries can be sustained over time, that is, if they fill up the block of time consistently. If block scheduling is not an option and the physician prefers to perform procedures at multiple locations, care should be taken to schedule him or her at one location for a minimum period of time.

One surgery office, for example, was struggling with scheduling surgeries and procedures at multiple locations. Often a physician was scheduled at three different locations in one morning. The practice solved the situation by scheduling the physician at one location once that location was first scheduled (i.e., if patient 1 wanted to go to location 1 on a particular Thursday, then patients 2, 3, and 4 who were scheduled for that Thursday would go to location 1). In addition, the physician agreed to visit two locations in the same day, effectively splitting the day in half between the two locations. This approach worked more smoothly than did the three-in-one-morning scheduling to which the surgeon was accustomed previously. Her production increased substantially.

Patients are often able to convince nursing staff that they need to be treated at one location as opposed to another. An assertive but kind nurse or scheduler who is able to steer patients to a particular location can be very beneficial in increasing physician productivity.

PRESCRIPTION DRUG PROGRAMS

Organization is needed to make sure patients have access to reduced prescription costs. Before Medicare started paying for medications in 2003, with the enactment of the Medicare Prescription Drug, Improvement, and Modernization Act, providing such access to patients was a more significant piece of nursing's responsibility. Nursing staff often tuck away forms and pamphlets related to reduced-cost medications given to them by pharmacy representatives, in case they are needed by a patient, but then they would have to search to find the materials when that once-a-year case came along.

Because a need still exists for medication assistance programs, organize a book in which nursing can promptly identify the right pharmaceutical company and give the patient the appropriate forms. This book becomes a reference source in helping patients. Once again, due to the complexity surrounding this task, one designated person may need to take on the role of disseminating reduced-cost drug information.

FMLA OR OTHER PAPERWORK

Patients hand the nursing staff all kinds of paperwork to be filled out for their employer, insurance company, or other stakeholder in the payment of their care. Such paperwork includes FMLA applications and disability claims. Having a clear policy on how to process these forms is important. In one practice, the nursing staff instructed patients carrying insurance forms or employer paperwork to return to the front desk after they were seen by the physician and to pay a nominal fee for the nursing staff to fill out the paperwork. At that time, the patient also completed a separate covering form providing relevant information, such as the items listed in **Exhibit 5.16**. The patient's covering form was then attached to the requested paperwork and placed on the nurse's desk, assuring the nurse that the paperwork had been handled by the front desk. The nurse was thus removed from the role of determining which type of paperwork required payment at the time of the visit and which did not, and how much that payment would be. The form was then filed in the chart in case additional questions arose.

Each type of paperwork could be analyzed to determine the right person to perform the task. Oftentimes, nursing expertise is not needed and a clerical staff can be asked to perform these actions.

EXHIBIT 5.16 Form Completion Request

We will be happy to complete any FMLA, disability or other miscellaneous forms that are required by your employer, insurance company, or other facility. There will be a charge of $ _____ for this service payable before the form is completed.

Please fill out the items below to assist us in completing your forms.

Today's Date _____

Patient name _____ Date of birth _____

Phone number _____ Physician _____

First day off work _____ Planned return to work _____

Signature _____

We will call you when your papers are ready for pickup. We can also fax them for you if you provide a fax number.

Please fax paperwork _____

Fax nunber _____

Thank you

PHARMACEUTICAL REPRESENTATIVES

If pharmaceutical representatives are not managed well, a major disruption will occur in patient flow. Most often the way into the practice for drug representatives is through the nursing staff. If the practice's nursing staff have a tendency to be timid or overly friendly, its physician may be inundated with pharmaceutical representative visits. The reality is that nursing staff control access to their physician. As with the other nursing aspects discussed in this chapter, a clear policy is needed for any practice, whether it declares "No drug reps" or defines specific times when drug representatives are allowed to visit. An example of one such policy is shown in **Exhibit 5.17**.

EXHIBIT 5.17 Pharmaceutical Representative Visits

1. Pharmaceutical representatives will be asked to sign in at the front desk and given a copy of this policy.

2. Only one pharmaceutical representative is allowed into the clinical area at a time.

3. Visits are limited to 10 minutes per visit and 1 minute per physician. Any staff member may ask the representative to finish his or her visit if the individual has overstayed the 10 minutes.

4. Some physicians may not have time to visit with the representative on a particular day. Nursing staff will inform the representative of this situation when he or she enters the clinical area.

5. If the representative has a new product or new information on a product that requires more than one minute of the physicians' time, a luncheon appointment should be scheduled.

6. Representatives will be stationed at _____ location in the clinical area. Staff should ask any representative to return to the specified area if he or she is found outside this area.

7. Representatives may leave any literature/new study material with one of the nursing staff for distribution to the physicians.

8. If a pharmaceutical representative does not follow the rules, the physicians may prohibit that representative from returning to the practice.

9. Stocking of samples can be done at any time. This activity is considered separate from the physician visit time.

10. A disposable container is available in the sample area for discarding outdated samples.

11. The representative will check back with the front desk staff to make them aware of the representatives leaving the practice.

12. Luncheons can be scheduled by calling the front office staff, who will schedule them in the luncheon book.

Also helpful in managing drug representative visits is providing assertive-response training. Knowing key assertive words and phrases can help staff control access. These representatives are salespeople who often can be difficult to curtail. If a policy is in place for dealing with them, the nurse can refer to it as a valid reason for "kicking them out."

QUALITY-OF-CARE STANDARDS / POPULATION HEALTH

Recent years have seen physicians being offered financial incentives by insurance companies to measure and achieve quality-of-care targets. Incentive-based performance improvement, or pay for performance and value-based reimbursement is experiencing an impressive rate of growth throughout the United States. The information technology needed to help physicians and nursing staff take advantage of all the latest data available on treatments, medications, risks, costs, and benefits, however, is not keeping the same pace. Nursing staff are now and will be a big part of measuring, reporting, and achieving quality-of-care measures. Improvement programs such as patient registries may be introduced into the practice to address quality-of-care concerns. Nursing staff input should be obtained in the implementation effort, as they are an important element in the patient care process.

Nursing may be involved in population health efforts through collecting, analyzing and correcting quality measures. Most of these measures involve the team and can be effectively influenced by posting of results for all to see. Discussion among teams and across teams in the most efficient way to document quality will lead to better outcomes. Determine who has the best practice with the best results and copy it.

PATIENT-CENTERED CARE

Quality nursing—including all aspects of the nursing role—is one key to patient-centered care in the medical office. This includes involving the patient in their care and always thinking about how your actions influence the patient. For example, a new policy might require you to put a patient bracelet on all patients so everyone knows they are a patient. However, that process may not be palatable to most patients since it puts a label on them as a patient instead of a person. The nurse's personality influences patients to return to the practice or to leave it. The nurse often is the person in the office who smooths an unpleasant experience with the reception staff, phone attendant, or physician. It is not uncommon, for example, to hear a nurse making excuses for a physician's behavior, whether it is related to his or her availability, abruptness, or personality. Sometimes, controlling damage incurred by another staff member can take up a significant part of the nurse's time. Conducting a continuous, open, and honest dialogue with the nursing staff, as well as providing education on patient centered care, can improve the nurse's effectiveness in dealing with patients.

PATIENT ENGAGEMENT

Patients who are informed are better engaged in their care. Include the patient as a team member, explaining all procedures and results. For example, the patient who knows their high cholesterol level can make a better choice on what food to eat or reject. Helping patients understand their illness and/or how to maintain a healthy lifestyle leads to a more involved patient.

CLINICAL TRIALS

The nurse may play a role in clinical trials management. He or she may be instrumental in identifying patients who qualify for a research study and may be the person who carries out the protocol for the clinical trial. If nursing staff are involved in clinical trials, they should have a full understanding of the process. This aspect of nursing is explained more fully in Chapter 10.

In summary, nursing is instrumental in many aspects of the practice. Helping the nurse become efficient in these areas reduces costs to the practice and results in satisfied patients and physicians.

Chapter 6

Supervision of Nursing Staff

One question that often arises related to practice management is whether both a nursing supervisor and a practice administrator are needed. The answer is not always clear. Some type of nursing supervisor is essential to provide clinical supervision of non-licensed staff. For large clinics, a midlevel manager provides management and guidance for the nursing staff because the administrator typically is unable to spend the time needed for adequate staff supervision and must delegate this responsibility. For smaller practices, the amount and type of supervisory positions depend on the particular needs and culture of the practice.

WHO SUPERVISES

Physicians provide guidance for the clinical staff members with whom they work: they instruct, give orders, and evaluate results of treatment. In short, they supervise the patient care provided to their patients. But do physicians supervise the staff? They certainly have the power to hire and fire by making their thoughts known they are—or should be—involved in staff evaluations, and they provide direction in clinical work functions. Physicians are leaders and should provide leadership to the clinical team, which includes feedback to team members and to supervisors. But most physicians prefer to have someone else in the practice provide overall supervision of their staff.

Some situations may require a clear definition of who is responsible for supervision. For example, one physician may want his nursing assistant to administer injections, and he intends to teach the assistant to do so. However, the clinic may have procedures and competency standards in place that are in conflict with the physician's wishes. If the nursing assistant administers the injection and the patient suffers an adverse event, the clinic's liability exposure increases..

A gray area emerges when licensed staff are employed at the practice. If the practice does not employ licensed staff, then clinical supervision is the responsibility of the physician. But if licensed staff are employed, any function related to nursing falls under the state's nurse practice act. In many states, all nursing activities, when performed by a non-licensed staff member, are performed under the supervision of a nurse. In other states, the physician is responsible for medical assistants and nurses might be responsible for nursing assistants. It is always prudent to consult and understand your state's nurse practice act.

Regardless, RNs spend considerable time studying and training to obtain their license, and they usually want to protect it. Therefore, they, as well as the practice, benefit from specific discussions and established procedures regarding delegating nursing duties. For further clarification, your state board of nursing should be consulted.

In practices that have designated clinical managers, the answer to who supervises clinical staff is fairly easy: the nursing supervisor. The physician may play a role, as mentioned earlier in the chapter, but ultimately the nursing supervisor maintains responsibility for all nursing actions.

DELEGATION

Most nursing functions can be delegated to staff with adequate training and demonstrated competence. Nursing functions should either be performed by a licensed staff member or be delegated to a non-licensed clinical staff member who is supervised in the performance of those functions.

Most boards of nursing address delegation of nursing duties in their state's nurse practice act. Even if a medical assistant falls under the supervision of the physician, delegation should be done effectively. Delegation requires the following from the delegating nurse/person:

- To assess the abilities of the person to whom the task is to be delegated,
- To train on the task,
- To verify competency, and
- To conduct follow-up evaluation

Accurately assessing others' abilities enables the nurse to determine if the person performing the delegated task can master it and, if not, what training is needed. One method of assessment is to administer a formal pretest if delegation is expected to occur frequently, such as with teaching medical assistants to give allergy shots. This pretest helps determine the learning needs of medical assistants so that training can be tailored to meet their needs.

Training of the task should include background information about the procedure to ascertain that the trained person understands the task fully. Background information for an injection task may include hand-washing techniques, reading a medication vial, or recognizing the medication's side effects. Training should make the delegated individual aware of all risks that may be encountered if the procedure is completed either correctly or incorrectly.

A competency check should be done in the presence of the trainer that includes the performance of the task. The results of this check should be documented. A follow-up check should then be done on a regular basis to ensure that the correct procedure is still being followed.

NEW EMPLOYEE TRAINING

A training program is a necessity for new employees that clarifies the expectations of the position and allows them to ask questions. It is not uncommon to see a new clinical employee start work at 9 a.m. and by 10 a.m. perform activities on his or her own. This situation is a disservice to both the current staff and the new employee and sets up the new employee for failure. Taking the time to train a new employee reaps benefits in the long run.

The type of training provided depends on the position in which the new employee has been hired, with many positions sharing training needs. For instance, all clinical staff will need to learn about state and federal Occupational Safety and Health Administration guidelines, safety procedures, and patient flow. In addition, the medical assistant will need a more detailed explanation of his or her role in rooming patients, documenting items in the patients' charts, or supply stocking. Orientation checklists, such as the one displayed in **Exhibit 6.1**, can be created for each position to aid in training new employees. The checklists do not replace a formal orientation but assist in making sure all necessary procedures are covered.

EXHIBIT 6.1 Orientation of New Nursing Staff

Employee name
Position
Start date
Basic orientation (time card, employee handbook, computer passwords, paperwork, phone orientation, HIPAA, OSHA, etc.) — see basic orientation sheet

Nursing orientation:

- Review of procedure book
- Tour of clinical and other areas
  - Exam room
  - Supply room
    - nursing
    - office
  - Nursing areas
  - Front desk
  - Physician offices
  - Medical records
- Review of paperwork requirements
  - Visit paperwork
  - Educational information
  - Charge sheets
  - Lab tests
  - Orders
- Equipment
  - Location
  - Sterilizer
  - EKG
  - Thermometer
  - Stethoscope
  - Portable O_2
  - Cardiac monitors
  - Pulse oximeter
  - Hyfrecator
- Patient flow
  - Follow other nursing staff
  - Review special procedures
  - Identify go-to person

Although creating a manual is time consuming, having one available that details each physician's preferences and procedures can be invaluable if his or her nurse leaves the practice or becomes indisposed. In addition to being a resource for the staff covering for the nurse, the manual also saves time when training a replacement. The manual can be as simple as a list of handwritten preferences updated as the physician identifies them (e.g., the nurse is expected to make sure that all breast cancer patients are undressed from the waist up).

COMPETENCY

While the nursing mantra is "see one, do one, teach one," the definition of competency can be characterized as "see one, do one, check one off." Competency is concerned with making sure the training that was provided is understood. This concept is particularly applicable to the education of unlicensed assistive personnel (UAP) because, most often, they have not undergone formal training. (Nursing staff typically undergo numerous competency checks throughout their educational process.)

Hospital nursing requires yearly competency checks for all nursing staff on various procedures. The validity of conducting competency checks in a medical office is questionable unless the size of the clinic is such that the cost and time spent administering them are spread over a large number of physicians. In this case, if testing yearly for competency is the only way to make sure that all clinical staff are performing their duties competently, then it should be implemented. However, in a small physician's office, the physician working side by side with staff will recognize pretty quickly if a competency issue is present.

If the practice is delegating nursing duties to unlicensed assistive personnel, a competency checklist should be included in the UAP's file. Many sources for competency checklists are available on the Internet. For example, the Centers for Disease Control and Prevention has developed numerous skills checklists for such procedures as injections and hand washing. A simple competency checklist created for an individual practice may look like the one presented in **Exhibit 6.2**.

Knowledge competency is also used in many clinics. So consider—is knowledge your staff possesses something you want them telling patients? Can you be assured that medical assistants or even nurses understand the lab tests they are teaching patients about? When thinking about competency, you might also think about how you verify accurate knowledge competency.

EXHIBIT 6.2 Competency Check: Subcutaneous Injections

Action	Met	Not Met	Date of Demonstration	Observer

1. Gathers supplies
 	
  i. medication
  ii. alcohol pad, needle, bandage, cotton ball				

2. Cleans off medication vial with alcohol				
3. Draws up medication using right dose				
4. Changes needle				
5. Selects injection sight				
6. Pinches up on tissue				
7. Inserts needle at 45-degree angle				
8. Injects medication				
9. Wipes off patient of any remaining blood				
10. Secures bandage				

ONGOING TRAINING

Each employee also must undergo training when changes in technique, process, or procedure are implemented, and so they remain up to date on new procedures or products. Ongoing training may be as simple as a 10-minute session at every nursing meeting, or bimonthly sessions on various topics. Continuous training is extremely helpful for UAPs in particular because it is a good way for them to gain more knowledge.

A yearly survey on training needs will document the gaps within the practice. The survey does not have to be formal, but input from staff is important to ensure the success of the training program. The content of programs should be both reactive (to meet current regulatory and process needs) and proactive (to meet growing external and internal expectations). At one surgery practice, surgeons each taught clinical staff a different surgical procedure so they would be more knowledgeable when talking with patients about the planned surgery. Not only was this approach tremendously beneficial to clinical staff, but it also helped the scheduler and the receptionist understand what the surgery actually entailed so they could schedule and route calls appropriately.

OVERALL SUPERVISION

Beyond clinical supervision, nonclinical managers can supervise the administrative aspects of nursing in a practice and do so successfully, just as clinical managers can successfully supervise nonclinical staff. The key to management of clinical staff by a non-clinician is for each party to recognize and accept that the nonclinical manager may not have a complete understanding of the activities in the nursing arena. A problem is created when nursing staff are led to believe that a non-clinician supervisor has expansive knowledge of the situations they are dealing with when he or she really does not. Honest and open communication can go a long way toward establishing a relationship between non-clinician supervisors and clinical staff. Have the nursing staff teach the nonclinical manager what obstacles impede their primary goal: taking care of patients. Most nurses are working in health care because they want to take care of patients rather than do paperwork or deal with insurance companies. Any measures taken to allow nursing staff to focus on patient care helps ease tensions related to knowledge of clinical operations.

There should always be a lead person in the practice who has a clinical mind-set, whether it is a nurse, lab technician, or physician. Clinical issues arise during the day that require someone's help in identifying and implementing solutions. Nursing staff often resolve issues among themselves, but they may need some assistance in complex situations. Having a clinically knowledgeable leader available to whom they can reach out in those situations will enable the clinic to continue to run smoothly.

MIDLEVEL MANAGEMENT

The use of a midlevel manager is more prevalent in larger clinics than in smaller offices. Clinical midlevel managers need basic management training such as in the following areas:

- Human resources principles
  - Interviewing and the hiring process
  - Managing separation/termination
  - Counseling
  - Performance management and evaluations

Discrimination

Harassment, including sexual harassment

Strategies for employee retention

Management principles

Problem solving

Time management

Strategic planning

Decision making

Financial principles

– Cost efficiency

– Budgeting at organizational level, at unit level, and for capital equipment

– Effective use of clinical resources

– Insurance funding

– Productivity

Leadership principles

Communication

Politics

Healthy work environments

Thinking as an organizational leader

Key attributes of a nurse leader

Leadership roles and responsibilities

Leading change

Staff development

Shared governance

Clinical management

Quality and outcomes

Patient care models

- Ensuring patient safety

- Strategies for managing a nursing department

- Ethics and social justice

- Disease management

- Medical practice demographics

- Personal and professional responsibility

  - Personal development and growth

  - Certification

  - Role negotiation

  - Career planning

This list is not all-inclusive, but is a start for any beginning clinical manager in a medical practice. All other factors being equal, hiring a seasoned manager is a better choice than hiring a novice, and managers with previous hospital clinical management experience typically bring added benefit to the practice. Both initial training, conducted with staff upon their employment, and ongoing training, conducted throughout their tenure with the practice, help clarify the nursing role.

Chapter 7

The Right Amount of Staff

Now that different issues relating to nursing staff, nursing functions, staff production measures, efficiency, and supervision of nursing staff have been addressed, how does a manager know the right number of staff to employ? Many ways are available to determine appropriate staffing levels. No one method is perfect, but when several are used in combination, a solid picture of staffing needs should emerge. Each practice's situation is different, and only the practice will know the right number of staff to get the job done.

BENCHMARKING

One of the easiest and fastest ways to assess staffing levels is to benchmark against other like practices. Benchmarking may be as easy as discussing staffing levels with a manager of a similar practice. Networking with other managers in the same specialty or in different specialties can lead to insight on how staffing is done at other practices.

A more formal way to benchmark is to work with an organization that compiles data relevant to staffing. Salary and benefits surveys are compiled by several organizations on both the local and national level. For example, the Medical Group Management Association's (MGMA) annual Cost Survey report benchmarks practices across the United States, dividing them by region, size, specialty, and ownership.[1]

---

1   Medical Group Management Association. 2008. Cost Survey for Single-Specialty Practices: 2008 Report Based on 2007 Data. Englewood, CO: Medical Group Management Association.

When benchmarking numbers are used, several considerations should be noted:

- the sample size is important
- a large sample provides a better representation of like practices, as a small sample may skew data in one direction or another
- regardless of the size, information may be gleaned from the data of other like practices
- and origin or location of data is important, as a practice serving a different section of the country may experience different utilization

Two terms used in comparison of similar practices are the mean and the median. The mean is the number reached by dividing a total (the sum of data items) by the number of data items. For example, say you are seeking the mean (average) of 10, 20, 30, 60, 65, and 70. Add the numbers from each item (255) and divide that sum by the number of items (6). The mean of these items is 42.5.

The median is simply the number that falls in the middle of an ordered list of values. Using the same example as above, the middle is between 30 and 60 (three numbers appear above the middle and three numbers appear below it), so the median is halfway between the two, or 45. Another term for the median is the 50th percentile.

The median provides a more accurate average because the existence of extremely high or extremely low values does not distort results, as may be the case with the mean.

MGMA's report is a good benchmark for medical practices because it gathers a high volume of national data for most specialties. With MGMA benchmarking, the first factors to consider are the number of reporting practices, the specialty of the practices, and the location of those practices.

MGMA staffing data are reported in terms of full-time-equivalent (FTE) physician or FTE provider (midlevel providers plus physicians) in mean and median averages. The median is reported in 10th percentile, 25th percentile, median or 50th percentile, 75th percentile, and 90th percentile. For each full-time physician in your practice, the 50th percentile of all like practices report the number indicated.

Consider the following example: A family practice has five physicians and three nurse practitioners. It employs six full-time registered nurses (RNs), five FTE licensed practical nurses (LPNs), and two full-time nursing assistants. (In actuality, it employs six LPNs total, but two work part time. One works two days per week [16 hours per week divided by 40 hours per week = 0.4 FTE], and one works three days per week [24 hours per week divided by 40 hours per week = 0.6 FTE].) An FTE in this practice works 40 hours per week.

EXHIBIT 7.1 FTE Staff		
	Family Practice FTE Staff	Family Practice Staff per FTE Physician
RN	6.0	1.2
LPN	5.0	1.0
NA/MA	2.0	0.4
Total clinical staff	13.0	2.60

In comparing this practice to MGMA-reported benchmarks, both individual classifications (RN, LPN, medical assistant/nursing assistant [MA/NA]) and clinical staff as a whole are examined.

EXHIBIT 7.2 FTE Staff per Provider			
	Family Practice FTE Staff	Family Practice Staff per FTE Physician	Family Practice Staff per Provider
RN	6.0	1.2	0.75
LPN	5.0	1.0	0.625
NA/MA	2.0	0.4	0.25
Total clinical staff	13.0	2.60	1.625

First, **Exhibit 7.1** breaks down the FTEs for this practice. The practice has 6.0 FTE nurses. Dividing these nursing FTEs by the five family practice physicians results in 1.20 FTE RNs for every FTE physician. Total clinical staff per FTE physician is 2.60. To calculate the FTE nursing staff by the total number of eight providers (five physicians, three nurse practitioners), each staff category is divided by 8, for 0.75 FTE RNs for every FTE provider. Total staff per FTE provider is 1.625. (See **Exhibit 7.2.**).

Next, compare this practice to the MGMA median for like family practice groups nationwide, shown in **Exhibit 7.3**. The initial impression gained by comparing this family practice to the MGMA data is that this practice may be overstaffed. Overall clinical staff for the family practice group per FTE physician is 2.60, compared with MGMA's 2.04. And the overall clinical staff per FTE provider is 1.625, compared with MGMA's 1.54. For individual classification of staff, more RNs and LPNs staff this practice than is the MGMA median, and fewer NA/MAs are employed by this family practice group than by other like practices reporting to MGMA. This practice's staffing mix is thus much different from the MGMA-reported median.

EXHIBIT 7.3 MGMA Comparison FTE per Physician Provider					
		By FTE Physician		By FTE Provider	
	Family Practice FTE Staff	Family Practice Staff per FTE Physician	MGMA Staff per FTE Physician	Family Practice Staff per FTE Provider	MGMA Staff per FTE Provider
RN	6.0	1.2	0.33	0.75	0.24
LPN	5.0	1.0	0.56	0.625	0.38
NA/MA	2.0	0.4	1.15	0.25	0.92
Total clinical staff	13.0	2.6	2.04	1.625	1.54

Source: Reprinted with permission from the Medical Group Management Association, 104 Inverness Terrace East, Englewood, Colorado 80112
877.ASK.MGMA www.mgma.com. Copyright 2008

Exhibit 7.4 shows a comparison of this practice's actual RN, LPN, and assistant staff FTEs to the FTEs demonstrated by the MGMA like practices. This comparison is obtained by multiplying the staff per FTE provider or physician by the number of physicians or providers (e.g., for RN: using physicians – $0.33 \times 5 = 1.65$ total staff; using providers – $0.24 \times 8 = 1.92$ total staff).

The practice appears to be overstaffed by approximately 0.68 FTE per provider (13.0 FTE compared with 12.32 FTE per MGMA FTE provider), but what is more evident is the result of the staffing mix comparison with MGMA: other like practices have 1.92 RNs, compared with 6.0 RNs at this family practice group. Similarly, other like practices have 7.36 FTE assistants, compared with this practice's 2.0 FTEs. This analysis shows that the family practice uses a costly staffing mix to ensure adequate coverage.

In the very first overview a practice conducts of how staffing compares with that in other like practices, a determination can be made immediately if the practice is staffed in alignment with other practices. Certainly, overstaffing may be justified in certain circumstances; for example, better-performing practices typically employ more staff.

EXHIBIT 7.4 MGMA Comparison by Number of Staff					
		By FTE Physician		By FTE Provider	
	Family Practice FTE Staff	MGMA Staff per FTE Physician	MGMA Total Staff Needed	MGMA Staff per FTE Provider	MGMA Total Staff Needed
RN	6.0	0.33	1.65	0.24	1.92
LPN	5.0	0.56	2.80	0.38	3.04
NA/MA	2.0	1.15	5.75	0.92	7.36
Total clinical staff	13.0		10.2		12.32

Source: Reprinted with permission from the Medical Group Management Association, 104 Inverness Terrace East, Englewood, Colorado 80112
877.ASK.MGMA www.mgma.com. Copyright 2008

DIFFERENCES AMONG SPECIALITIES

As implied at the outset of this chapter, differences exist among the practices of various specialties. Family practice providers need more staff than orthopedic providers, for example. To exemplify the impact of differences between specialties on staffing, consider the following example: Assume an orthopedic practice has the same staff as the family practice used in the previous example (six RNs, five LPNs, and two NAs/MAs). Use the MGMA Cost Survey numbers for like orthopedic practices to analyze this practice's staffing, shown in **Exhibit 7.5**.

EXHIBIT 7.5 MGMA Comparison by Different Speciality

	Orthopedic FTE Staff	Orthopedic Staff per FTE Physician	MGMA Staff per FTE Orthopedic Physician	MGMA Total Staff Needed for Orthopedic Physician	MGMA Total Staff Needed for Family Practice Physician *
RN	6.0	1.2	0.33	1.65	1.65
LPN	5.0	1.0	0.37	1.85	2.80
NA/MA	2.0	1.4	0.84	4.20	5.75
Total clinical staff	13.0	2.6	1.54	7.70	10.2

* from Exhibit 7.4
Source: Reprinted with permission from the Medical Group Management Association, 104 Inverness Terrace East, Englewood, Colorado 80112
877.ASK.MGMA www.mgma.com. Copyright 2008

When comparing the staffing needs of a family practice with those of an orthopedic practice using the MGMA medians, the difference is 2.5 FTE nursing staff (10.2 for family practice compared with 7.7 for orthopedic).

USING THE MEASURES

Chapter 4 identifies many different measures to analyze staff production. Here, using similar examples, staffing need is demonstrated. For this example, the same family practice group used in the example above is analyzed in terms of provider visit data, shown in **Exhibit 7.6**.

The visits are broken down by week and by day of the week. The totals for all providers on that day are shown in each line item, which represents a week of time for three months. Totals are shown at the bottom of the first table and then averaged in the middle of the exhibit. The averages reflect only those days on which physicians saw patients and exclude vacation and holiday time. For example, the average visit volume for the 15-week period for Monday clinics was 100 patients. Below the averages, the visit numbers are listed by type of clinical staff for eight providers. The x represents a nursing staff member present and working. For those 100 patients coming through the practice on Monday, for instance, 13 nursing staff were working.

Exhibit 7.6 Average Visits per Day

Week	M	Tu	W	Th	F
1		105	103	102	51
2	94	107	83	45	0
3	60	70	51	61	37
4	79	89	83	81	45
5	127	109	97	80	0
6	67	69	96	80	62
7	118	114	93	70	42
8	96	123	98	77	37
9	146	116	92	85	60
10	103				
11		91	79	93	21
12	122	109	69	87	49
13	83	73	68	69	43
14	112	150	100	101	35
15	92	88	86	68	
Total	1,299	1,413	1,198	1,099	482
	M	Tu	W	Th	F
Average	100	101	86	79	44
RN					
One	x	x	x	x	x
Two	x	x	x	x	x
Three	x	x	x	x	x
Four	x	x	x	x	x
Five	x	x	x	x	x
Six	x	x	x	x	x
	6	6	6	6	6
LPN					
One	x	x			
Two	x	x	x	x	x
Three	x	x	x	x	x
Four			x	x	x
Five	x	x	x	x	x
Six	x	x	x	x	x
	5	5	5	5	5
CNA					
One	x	x	x	x	x
Two	x	x	x	x	x
Total	2	2	2	2	2

The results seem to indicate that too many nursing staff are assisting with physician office visits. At this point in the analysis, it can be determined that the practice may have employed too many nursing staff for its needs, but let us delve further into the analysis to validate that finding.

Phone call volume for this practice was heavy, as the table of incoming calls shown in **Exhibit 7.7** demonstrates.

The table is broken down by day of week and time of call for a two-week period. Total phone calls and average phone calls are calculated, as are percentage of calls by time of day. All Monday phone calls are totaled and divided to arrive at an average phone call volume for Mondays. The averages of 630 phone calls on Monday, 570 on Tuesday, 501 on Wednesday, 500 on Thursday, and 276 on Friday—a much lighter call-volume day than that of the other days of the week—may signify opportunities for streamlining staffing and increasing efficiency if studied in detail.

Next, nursing procedures were analyzed over a two-month period for walk-in patients and included allergy and other injections, stress tests, electrocardiograms (EKGs), and Holter monitor placement procedures. These represented a significant proportion of the nursing procedures performed at this clinic. The table shown in **Exhibit 7.8** demonstrates the procedure numbers per month for the two-month time period.

Once again, the numbers of each procedure type were calculated on a per-month basis and a two-month average was determined. This number was then divided by four (4) to determine, on average, how many procedures were performed each day of the week (e.g., injections: 285 first month + 248 second month = 533 ÷ 2 = 267 ÷ 4 = 67 injections performed every Monday, on average).

After gathering data on the different components being studied, the next step is to combine the above visit volume, phone call volume, and nursing visit volume and make a staffing determination (**Exhibit 7.9**). For purposes of this example, assumptions are made on how many visits an FTE can room, how many phone calls an RN can manage, and how many procedures an FTE can perform. The actual numbers will be clinic specific and depend on demographics of the patient base. (The ability of the nursing staff should not be considered when determining these number because some nurses work slower and less efficiently than others. A time study to determine the appropriate number of procedures and/or phone calls can provide an approximate benchmark.)

EXHIBIT 7.7 Phone Call Volume

Date	1	4	5	6	7	8	11	12	13	14	Totals	Avg	%
	F	M	Tu	W	Th	F	M	Tu	W	Th			
Incoming Calls													
Before 9 a.m.	39	48	38	33	37	46	65	42	40	28	416	42	7
9-10 a.m.	55	87	81	46	56	58	69	73	49	52	626	63	11
10-11 a.m.	68	72	75	64	71	56	69	50	53	41	619	62	11
11-12 noon	62	68	53	76	55	56	61	65	51	42	589	59	11
12-1 p.m.	68	40	23	22	30	44	54	36	39	38	394	44	8
1-2 p.m.		64	74	81	66		73	60	68	62	548	69	12
2-3 p.m.		61	61	63	47		65	75	65	58	495	62	11
3-4 p.m.		72	41	56	48		58	74	51	61	461	58	10
4-5 p.m.		81	74	48	55		70	50	56	75	509	64	11
After 5 p.m.		26	64	22	44		57	30	19	34	296	37	7
	292	619	584	511	509	260	641	555	491	491	4,953	557	99

Average Calls Per Day

	Total	Avg	%
Monday	1,260	630	25
Tuesday	1,139	570	23
Wednesday	1,002	501	20
Thursday	1,000	500	20
Friday	552	276	11
	2,477		99

Note: Percentages do not equal 100 due to rounding

EXHIBIT 7.8 Nursing Visits

	Month 1					Month 2				
Nursing Visits	M	Tu	W	Th	F	M	Tu	W	Th	F
Allergy shot	50	25	96	76	50	28	38	80	67	57
Injection	235	386	352	543	501	220	253	566	371	325
Total	285	411	448	619	551	248	291	646	438	382
1-month average	267	351	547	529	466					
Daily average	67	88	137	132	117					
OB stress	17	4	16	39	5	1	44	17	31	10
EKG	47	46	55	84	62	50	40	43	99	56
Stress	30	8	34	30	18	20	4	37	36	26
Holter	10	0	7	11	6	7	2	14	13	12
Total	104	58	112	164	91	78	90	111	179	104
1-month average	91	74	112	172	98					
Daily average	23	19	28	43	25					

Exhibit 7.9 Nursing Visits, Phone Calls, Visits Summary

	M	Tu	W	Th	F	Total
Visits per day	100	101	86	79	44	
If 30 visits per FTE staff to room patients	**3.33**	**3.37**	**2.87**	**2.63**	**1.47**	
Phone calls	630	570	501	500	276	
If 150 calls per FTE staff	**4.20**	**3.80**	**3.34**	**3.33**	**1.84**	
Nursing visits						
Injections	67	88	137	132	117	
Testing	23	19	28	43	25	
If 30 procedures per day per FTE staff	**3.00**	**3.57**	**5.50**	**5.83**	**4.73**	
Total staff needed	**10.53**	**10.74**	**11.71**	**11.79**	**8.04**	

Note: Italic denotes totals; bold denotes FTEs needed to staff the number of visits.

On Monday, on average, 100 provider visits and 630 phone calls were encountered, and 67 injections and 23 tests were performed. Assuming that one nurse can handle 30 provider visits, one nurse can handle 150 phone calls, and one nurse can handle 30 procedures, then a total of 10.53 FTE staff are needed on Monday. Looking at the other days of the week, staffing needs vary from 8 to 12 FTEs depending on the day. Taking into consideration all these data, the family practice's nursing staff total of 13 may be too high if 13 staff work every day.

Because we do not know what nursing responsibilities are included for those practices reporting to MGMA, it is important to conduct further analysis of your practice. The duties are probably similar for other like practices, and the difference may occur in the efficiency of staff or processes. In another practice, one nurse may be able to handle 200 phone calls per day or 50 procedures per day. Therefore, viewing staffing in several different ways can lead to a determination based on subjective (practice demographics) and objective (MGMA benchmarks) data.

EXHIBIT 7.10 Hours Not Directly Assigned to Provider			
	June	July	August
RN1	96	108	88
2	160	176	176
3	8	24	24
4	52	40	28
5		26	34
6	32	36	40
LPN1	36	28	12
2	4		28
3	28	12	18
4	28	24	28
5,6	24	24	48
MA1	20	40	26
2	16	32	40
Total hours not assigned to provider	504	570	590
Total hours available per month FTE	160	176	176
FTEs not assigned to provider	**3.15**	**3.30**	**3.35**

Toward this end, we explore whether and how often nursing staff are performing other tasks besides working directly with physicians. Examining hours not directly assigned to a provider can give an indication of the scope of other duties performed in this practice (**Exhibit 7.10**) to supplement data regarding phones and procedures.

EXHIBIT 7.11 Overtime (OT) in 13-Week period		
	OT Total	Weeks with OT
RN1	20.29	5
2	19.4	7
3	12.8	5
4	7.67	2
5	22.21	4
6	1.86	5
LPN1	27.59	6
2	11.57	2
3	11.56	4
4	7.32	3
5	0	
6	0	
NA1	30.85	9
2	25.37	10
Total overtime	198.49	

This review considers those hours that nursing staff were not assigned to a provider. Some downtime not working with a provider is expected, and the totals reflect the extent of that downtime as well as the time spent by those nursing staff performing procedures and phone triage. The table breaks down the hours spent by each RN, LPN, and MA. Hours during which these nursing staff were not assigned to a provider seeing patients in the office were recorded. For each month of a three-month period, the number of total hours of all staff was divided by 160 hours (40 hours per week × 4 weeks) to arrive at a value representing an FTE not assigned to a provider.

Calculating this time is important in conjunction with viewing phone triage and nursing procedures. Recall that **Exhibit 7.9** demonstrates that in this practice, the nursing staff fielded 630 phone calls on Monday, and it was calculated that

4.20 FTE staff were needed. Similarly, for the procedures performed on Monday, 3.0 FTE nursing staff were needed.

Because staff share responsibilities in this practice, viewing the data in several ways, as shown in this chapter, assists in determining appropriate staffing. Obviously, staff assigned to providers were also providing phone triage and performing nursing visits. Opportunities to improve nursing staff organization to gain efficiency could be determined from these data.

A final factor considered at this practice was the use of overtime (**Exhibit 7.11**). Overtime usage can be attributed to too much work or to poor time management.

With the staffing situation already indicating overstaffing on many levels, the results of the overtime analysis, seen in **Exhibit 7.11**, are surprising. Some opportunities in time management and operational efficiency are definitely available that could assist this practice.

In summary, many measures can be used to help determine appropriate clinical staffing in a medical practice. One measure—benchmarking data—can immediately reveal if the practice is overstaffed. However, extenuating circumstances may have created this overstaffing. For the practice profiled here, the phone call volume is significant, as is the procedure volume. In this example, total visit numbers, phone calls, and procedure visit numbers were examined. The next step to determine appropriate staffing for this office is to analyze individual duties of each staff member and to determine which duties require an RN, an LPN, or an MA. The staffing model may be the problem at this practice, as discussed in the next section; the raw numbers give only part of the answer. Looking at the individual practice roles and responsibilities adds clarity to overall staffing analysis. Management should seek opportunities to assist the nursing staff to become more efficient. As a result of these efforts, staffing needs may be reduced over time.

NURSING MODELS

Nursing staff can be employed in many ways in a hospital and, by extension, in the community setting. This section considers the most common nursing models used in hospitals over the last few decades and shows their adaptation to the medical office. A practice may introduce variations on how each of these models is used. In the end, if the model works for the practice, then it is the right one.

For a better understanding of nursing model variations, we look at a family physician office of five physicians and two midlevel providers.

PRIMARY NURSING OR TOTAL PATIENT CARE

One of the best models of patient care for hospitals is primary care nursing (**Exhibit 7.12**). However, it is also the most expensive. Primary nursing has the following characteristics:

- It is usually entirely composed of RN staff.

- Each RN is fully responsible for patient care.

- Nurses have high autonomy and responsibility.

- The patient receives holistic and unfragmented care (i.e., one RN performs all care).

- The integral role of the primary nurse is to establish communication among the physician, the patient, and other team members.

- Other team members may include associate RNs, who provide patient care under the direction of the RN.

- Disadvantage—the high cost of RN wages.

EXHIBIT 7.12 Primary Nursing: Hospital

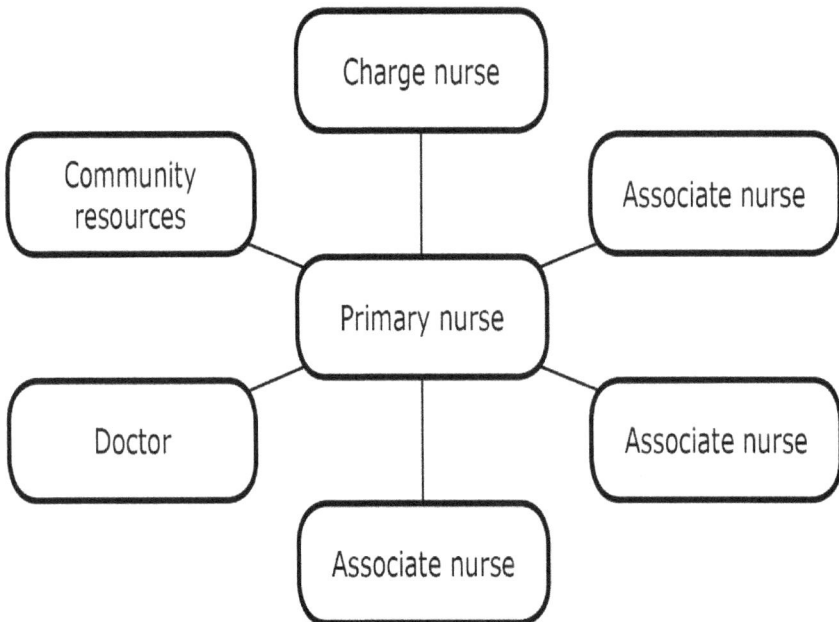

Although very effective in hospitals, this model is seldom used in medical practices due to the high cost. While the key to primary nursing is the use of an RN for all patient care, variations of this approach may be present in practices, whereby the physician may have nursing staff assigned to him or her only (**Exhibit 7.13**). The nursing staff member may be a nurse, an LPN, or a medical assistant whose primary duty is to room patients, teach patients, and manage telephone calls from patients for that physician.

EXHIBIT 7.13 Primary Nursing: Medical Practice

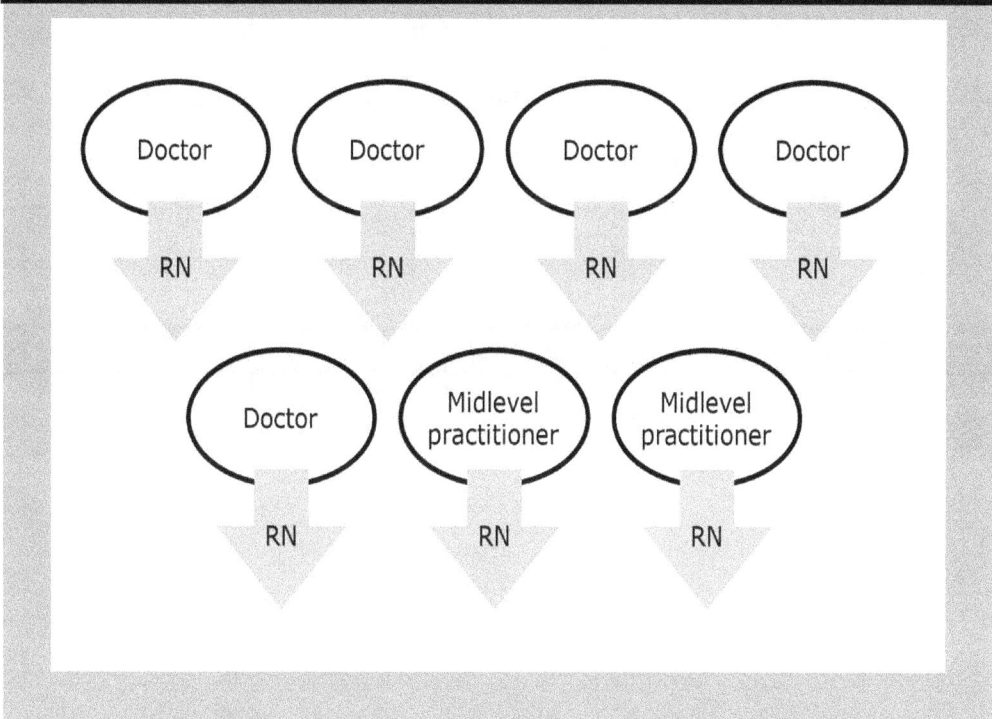

As with hospital-based primary nursing, the cost of this nursing care model is the highest for any practice. Actual RN cost varies, however, depending on practice location or specialty. **Exhibit 7.14** calculates a typical cost breakdown for primary nursing in a practice.

EXHIBIT 7.14 Cost of Primary Nursing

7 RNs @ $25/hour
@ $52,000 per RN=
$364,000 + benefits

TEAM NURSING

To offset declining reimbursements in hospitals, the team nursing concept was developed, whereby the RN is used exclusively for those tasks that require his or her expertise and license, and supporting tasks are assigned to other members of the team (**Exhibit 7.15**). Characteristics of team nursing include the following:

- Personnel working together to provide care for a group of patients under the direction of the RN,

- Extensive team communications,

- Small team providing care,

- Autonomy and shared responsibility and accountability, and

- High proportion of staff involved.

- Disadvantages—improper implementation, insufficient time for team planning and communication.

EXHIBIT 7.15 Team Nursing: Hospital

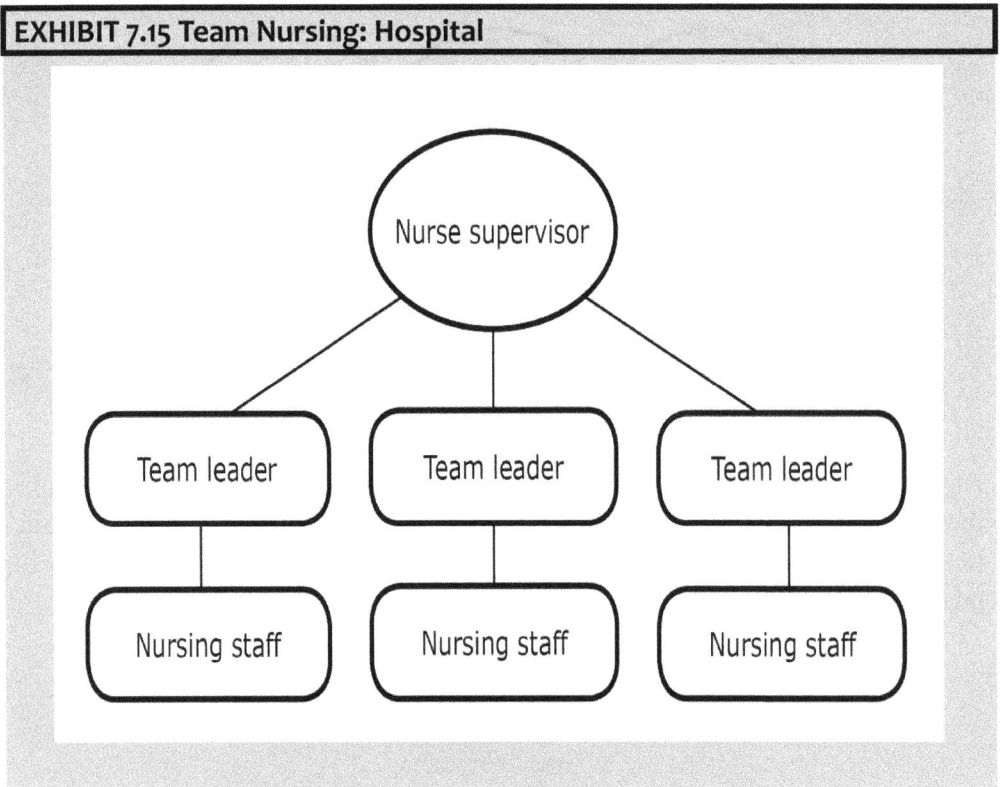

In a medical office, this nursing model can be useful and cost effective (**Exhibit 7.16**). For example, the RN will be used for phone triage and teaching, and the unlicensed assistive personnel will be used to room patients, stock supply rooms, and assist the RN as needed.

EXHIBIT 7.16 Team Nursing: Medical Office

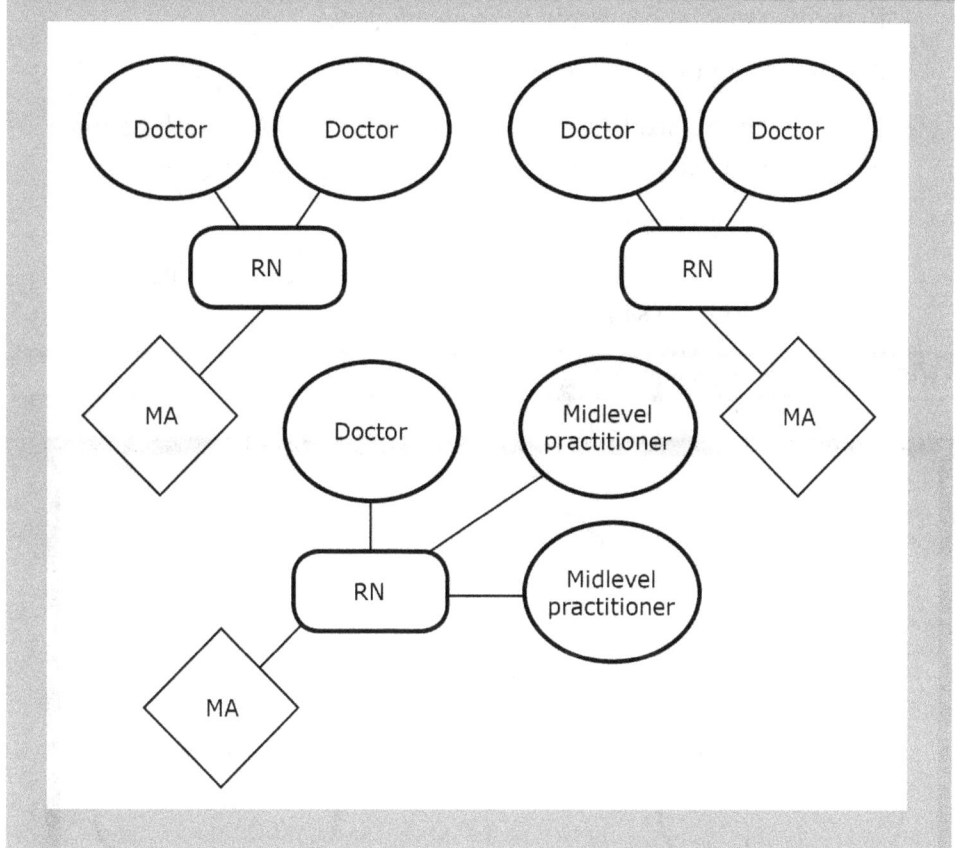

The cost effectiveness of this approach is apparent in the analysis shown in **Exhibit 7.17** (compare with the primary nursing cost breakdown in **Exhibit 7.14**).

EXHIBIT 7.17 Cost of Team Nursing

3 RNs @ $25/hour	$ 52,000	per year X 3 =	$	156,000
3 MAs @ $14/hour	$ 29,120	per year X 3 =	$	87,360
Total		$243,360 + benefits		

FUNCTIONAL NURSING

For maximum efficiency, nursing staff can be assigned certain tasks to perform for a group of patients (**Exhibit 7.18**). Characteristics of this approach are the following:

- Specific tasks are assigned to certain individuals.
- Repetitive motion occurs, increasing efficiency.
- A minimal number of registered nurses are needed.
- Training is provided to non-RN clinical staff on simple task performance (e.g., checking blood pressures, bathing, stocking supplies).
- Advantage—greater efficiency.
- Disadvantages—fragmented care, possibility of overlooking patient needs, and low job satisfaction.

EXHIBIT 7.18 Functional Nursing

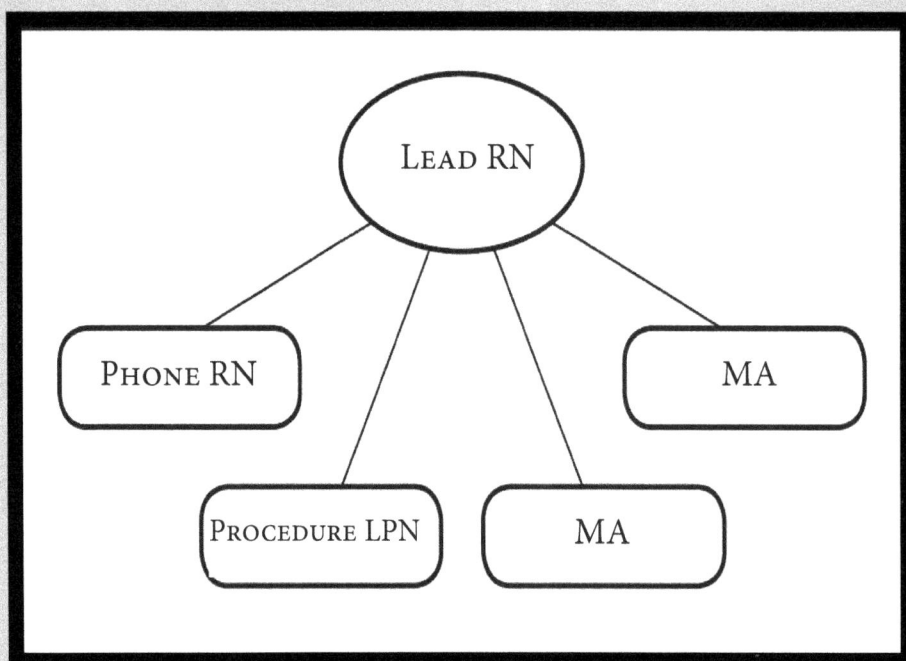

This model works well in primary care. Assignments may be set up in the following manner: MAs to room patients, RNs to cover telephone management, LPNs to perform procedures and medication administration, and lead nurse to help wherever needed. The cost of the functional nursing model in physician practices is much lower than that related to primary nursing and team nursing (**Exhibit 7.19**).

EXHIBIT 7.19 Cost of Functional Nursing

Lead RN + Phone RN			
(2 RN) @ $25/hour	$ 52,000	per year X 2 =	$ 104,000
1 LPN @ $19/hour	$ 39,520	per year X 1 =	$ 39,520
2 MAs @ $14/hour	$ 29,120	per year X 2 =	$ 58,140
Total			Benefits + $201,760

Other models of care are emerging in nursing and in health care in general. The clinical ladder model, for example, involves several different levels of nursing care, helps determine performance expectations, and recognizes work done at a specific level. It provides direction for staff in development and education as they move from level to level. Each successive level identifies increasing clinical proficiency skills and performance standards. Clinical ladders are usually seen in practices that clearly delineate roles and use professional nurses. The clinical ladder model can be implemented in conjunction with other models.

Another nursing model is case management. This approach is seen more in treatment of specific populations of patients. The nurse acts as an advocate to manage the patient's care. He or she coordinates all care for one patient or a group of patients. Most often this model is used to contain costs in chronic illness cases.

An emerging trend in nursing and performance improvement in hospitals is the Magnet designation. Three features of Magnet status are (1) professional autonomy over one's practice; (2) nursing control over the practice environment; and (3) effectiveness of communication among nurses, physicians, and administration.[2] How the Magnet program will affect nursing care in medical practices is still unclear.

---

2   Seago, Jean. 2001. "Nurse Staffing, Models of Care Delivery, and Interventions."www.ahrq.gov/clinic/ptsafety/chap39.htm. (Accessed 11/15/08.)

PATIENT-CENTERED MEDICAL HOME

In primary care practices, the patient-centered medical home model focuses on the ongoing physician-patient relationship with the care team in managing the entire panel of patients through coordination of both preventive and chronic disease care. Better access to care and information, population health, team based care and care management allow for better patient management. As this model develops, it has had an impact on nursing care in a medical office One main area of impact is team-based care and how nursing roles are emerging such as care managers, care coordinators and health coaches. We are seeing the true value of nursing as medical offices are reframing their team structure and roles.

There are many ways to look at clinical staffing needs. The primary goal is to provide quality care at the lowest possible cost to the practice. Quality care will differ by practice. Identifying your staffing needs allows you to move forward with staffing decisions. This author does not advocate replacing RNs with MAs. However, if you have a staffing vacancy, opportunities to improve efficiency and cost should be explored. It may take years to achieve the optimal staffing level and mix, but knowing where you should be is the first step in getting there.

Chapter 8

Clinical Supply Resources

One of the main nursing functions in any medical clinic is management of resources. This area of responsibility includes managing all supplies, from medications to medical forms, used for the patient visit. All practices use supplies of some sort, some more than others. This chapter focuses on management of medications, medical supplies, equipment, forms, and patient education materials.

PHARMACEUTICAL SUPPLIES

The types of medications kept in the practice vary from clinic to clinic. A primary care clinic may keep as many as 40 different medications in stock, whereas a surgical practice may keep fewer than five. Drug samples may constitute a large part of an oncology clinic, whereas an orthopedic practice may have no samples at all. Medications can be obtained from different sources, from the local pharmacy to medical supply vendors. Often a physician's signature is needed to initiate the one-time order or repeat ordering through a vendor. The task of maintaining adequate medication supplies should be assigned to one individual for consistency and to maximize cost savings.

SAMPLES

Continued high prescription costs may prevent the patient from filling a prescription. The use of drug samples provided to the practice by pharmaceutical representatives helps initiate treatment and assists the patient financially. However, the use of samples can pose a liability threat if the drug's expiration date has passed, if patients are not given adequate education about the drug, or if staff avail themselves of the sample closet.

Management of the sample supply should include controlling access to storage cabinets and prohibiting the use of samples without instructions and/or permission from a provider. It is not uncommon for staff to self-medicate if the sample closet is easily accessible; obtaining free medication samples may even be considered by some staff to be a benefit of working in a clinic setting. However, only providers should prescribe or direct the use of sample medications. Some clinic situations may require even stricter controls. Putting a straightforward procedure in place regarding drug samples clarifies expectations for staff. If, for example, the sample supply cabinet is located in a busy, high-traffic area, staff abuse may be mitigated.

Patients should not have access to samples. Placing sample medications in examination rooms away from the eyes of staff should be avoided. When samples are given to patients, written instructions with medication, strength, dose, and frequency should accompany the samples to ensure their proper use. A log can be kept in the sample closet to track usage of samples or to provide assistance in locating patients who took the sample if a medication recall occurs.

Organizing the sample closet to maximize ease in locating the right sample can increase efficiency for both staff and physicians. Using storage bins that are clearly labeled and arranged by drug classification (e.g., allergy medication, antibiotics) simplifies the task of retrieving samples. The organization method used should be clear to those responsible for stocking the closet. Some practices allow vendors to stock the cabinets, thereby saving staff time. This procedure should not be a problem as long as storage containers are clearly marked. Placing the newest stock in the back of the storage container and the oldest in the front may reduce or eliminate storage of expired drug samples. Expiration dates should be checked on a regular basis, and outdated samples should be discarded in a safe manner—usually in a biohazard container kept in the sample closet, not in the regular trash container. Vendors may take expired drugs out of the practice if they assist with stocking.

A samples procedure may be included as a part of your overall medication procedure. An example of the samples portion of a medication procedure is shown in **Exhibit 8.1**.

ORAL, TOPICAL, AND INJECTABLE MEDICATIONS

Oral medication may not be as common in clinics as is injectable medication, but in certain situations it may be needed (e.g., anti-emetic tablets in oncology, nitroglycerin tablets in an internal medicine office). Oral medication may be packaged in individually wrapped packets or in a multidose vial. Topical medications may also be kept in the practice (e.g., nitroglycerin paste). Controls regarding these medications should be the same as those regarding sample medications, including attention to location, storage, rotation, checking for outdates, and so forth.

EXHIBIT 8.1 Samples Procedure

Location and Organization
- Samples will be located _____.
- Samples will be organized according to classification of medication and then alphabetically:

– Antibiotics	– Gastric motility
– Antidepressants	– Hormone replacement
– Antihistamines	– Hyperlipidemia
– Arthritis	– Migraine
– Cardiac/hypertension	– Pain medications
– Contraception	– Pulmonary
– Diabetic	

- Samples will be checked weekly for outdated items.
- When stocked, samples with new expiration dates will be placed in the back.
- Patients will not have access to the sample closet.
- Samples can be discarded in a biohazard box placed in the sample closet.

Physician Order
- Samples will be dispensed only under the direction of a physician.
- Staff wanting samples will go through a physician or his or her nurse to obtain samples.

Patient Instructions
- Patients will be given clear instructions when provided sample medications, including:
    - Medication name—make sure patient is aware of generic or brand name, if different
    - Dosage and frequency
    - Route—by mouth, rectal, etc.
    - Major side effects—may cause drowsiness, dry mouth, etc.
    - Specific instructions with medication—take with food, take on empty stomach, do not take with milk products, etc.
- Patients should be given enough samples to manage their condition and/or enable them to obtain a filled prescription. Amount is under the direction of the physician.

Multidose or single-use injectable medications are often used in primary care clinics as well as in oncology, orthopedics, and other specialty practices. Upon opening any multidose vial medication, it is important to date and initial the vial.

This author recommends keeping open vials no longer than 30 days. However, most sources do not clearly state when an open vial should be discarded.

Controlling access to injectable medications, as with other medications, is necessary. Injectable medications, especially immunizations, can be very costly. As suggested above, a log may be kept to document injectable medication usage for more controlled access. Some injectable medications require refrigeration. Be sure to check the label for any such instructions. (See also the section on vaccines below.)

As with other medications, the stocking and ordering process for injectable medications should include discarding expired drugs on a regular basis in the biohazard box.

NARCOTICS

Federal law requires the control of any U.S. Drug Enforcement Administration Schedule drug or narcotic by limiting access in a locked cabinet or drawer. Counts of each narcotic should occur after each shift, or daily, and be carried out by two individuals. **Exhibit 8.2** is an example of a log used for this function.

A separate log is created for each medication that needs to be monitored. As shown in the exhibit, the medication name and initial supply number are listed. After each removal from the locked location, the medication and the name of the patient the medication is given to are listed on the log, with the quantity given, the supply remaining, and any additions (e.g., more medication added) or subtractions (e.g., medication given to another practice). At the end of the shift, each sheet is reviewed to ensure it matches the inventory.

EXHIBIT 8.2 Narcotics Log

Medication _____   Initial Supply _____

Patient and Dose Given (e.g.,50 mcg)	Quantity Given (e.g., 1 vial)	Supply Remaining	Additions/ Subtractions

VACCINES

Vaccines are stored differently from other injectable medications and are often refrigerated. Recommended temperatures specific to vaccines are available from the Centers for Disease Control and Prevention (CDC).[1] Vaccines that require refrigeration need a dedicated place for their storage; food and beverages should not be stored in the same unit. Thermometers in the vaccine storage area should also be used to ensure the proper temperature is maintained.

INTRAVENOUS MEDICATIONS

Intravenous stock is used in oncology, cardiology, and other specialty practices. These medications can be ordered premixed or can be mixed at the practice. Mixing drugs may require the use of a protective hood. Check with the CDC or a pharmacist to ensure compliance with regulatory requirements.

Intravenous flushes for central lines most often come as multiuse vials and should be dated and initialed when opened. They can also be ordered in single-use vials, which eliminate potential contamination issues and may increase efficiency. Individual flushes may be prepared from a multidose vial daily. Make sure they are properly labeled so no confusion arises as to what the solution is and when it was prepared.

Use of the patient's personal medication supplies, especially in oncology or at urgent care centers, should be limited. Often, patients are encouraged to bring their own supplies to the visit to assist the nurse and to reduce costs. Ensuring the validity of personal products requires the presence of an intact, unopened vial for administration in the clinic setting.

PRESCRIPTION PADS

Although e-prescribing is prevalent in most offices, some office still have a supply of prescription pads. It should be guarded closely and kept out of sight and away from the access of patients. Some physicians want to keep prescription pads in the exam rooms for convenience, but providing patients such easy access to them is strongly discouraged. Most patients will not take an accessible prescription pad for his or her own use, but allowing patients the opportunity invites that illegal activity.

A strict policy on who can call prescriptions in to the pharmacy should also be in place. Frequently reported nursing violations of the state nurse practice act include cases in which a nurse writes a prescription and/or calls in a prescription for himself or herself. Any nurse who performs an act of practicing medicine

---

1   Centers for Disease Control and Prevention. 2014. "Vaccine Storage and Handling Toolkit." (Accessed 2/28/2016.) http://www.cdc.gov/vaccines/recs/storage/toolkit/storage-handling-toolkit.pdf

violates the state's nurse practice act, and the practice manager is required to report the incident to the state board of nursing.

OSHA-MANDATED REQUIREMENTS

Any liquid medication used in the practice requires an accompanying Material Safety Data Sheet to be kept available to staff as a reference according to Occupational Safety and Health Administration regulations. Chapter 10 provides more information about this topic.

MEDICAL SUPPLIES

Medical supplies are used during most office visits. Nursing is responsible for maintaining supplies in the examination rooms, procedure rooms, and stock room. The quantity and location of each supply are important considerations when determining supply needs. For example, is it necessary for each of your 20 exam rooms to have 10 large ABD dressings, 20 4×4 dressings, and 20 2×2 dressings in its storage cabinet? Depending on how often the rooms are used, it may be necessary. More likely, the staff have placed that amount of supplies in the room so that stocking can be done less often. Developing a list of supplies that should be stocked in each room allows anyone to stock during downtime. Stocking duties are usually delegated to non-licensed staff and are often the last activity performed on a given shift. Stocking must take higher priority than it typically does, and it should be performed consistently according to a schedule each day.

The approach taken to stocking rooms is usually based on what supplies the physician uses during each visit. In some practices, physicians share rooms due to space considerations. If there is a chance that nursing staff or physicians may work in more than one exam room, then each room should be stocked in a similar fashion, as discussed in Chapter 5. In any specialty practice, the situation may arise in which a physician decides to add an office visit at the last minute to accommodate a patient, but another physician is using his regular exam room. Because common items are used during each visit, one container or specific drawer can be designated for these items so that the physician who moves to a different room will know exactly where to find the common items. A basic list of supplies in this container might include the items shown in **Exhibit 8.3**.

Using a consistently applied system and identifying one person for ordering supplies can eliminate the frustration resulting from being without a needed item at any given time. Usually, in smaller clinics, one of the nursing staff takes on this responsibility. In larger clinics, supplies are typically maintained by a separate department. Selecting the right person for this job is crucial to controlling costs of medical supplies. Say, for instance, that in an urgent care setting of a multispecialty clinic, every physician wants to use a different kind of suture. If every type were stocked, up to 50 different kinds of suture may be on hand in the supply closet. Is it really necessary to have so many different, expensive sutures whose expiration date will soon pass? Probably not. A good supply person should identify 8 to 10 different suture types and seek agreement from all the physicians that no more will be ordered unless agreed on by all.

EXHIBIT 8.3 Basic List of Supplies	
Dressings	Other
• 6 gauze 4x4-inch dressings	• 3 sterile cotton applicators
• 6 Telfa 2x2-inch dressings	• 6 tongue depressors
• 3 ABD pads	• 3 paper measuring tapes
• 3 gauze 2x2-inch dressings	• 12 alcohol prep pads
• 1 box of Bandaid -type bandages	• 3 betadine swabsticks
• 6 steri strips	• 2 of each syringes 10 cc, 5 cc

If a physician wants a new gadget or supply, an established procedure should be followed for approving its order prior to the order being placed. Some physicians might balk at having to follow a procedure to obtain a supply. However, the procedure is critical for determining supply needs. Sometimes it is necessary to order that once-in-a-lifetime product; the key is making sure that both the physician and the supply clerk think through the process prior to ordering.

A consistent system may include a chalkboard or grocery-style list placed in a key location to identify items needed. When a nursing staff member takes the last item of a supply, he or she writes down the item for replenishment. Designating a trash can for all empty supply boxes can serve as a place for the supply clerk to check for reordering, especially if the use of specialty items varies.

Supply ordering can be performed in numerous ways, including in person, online, or by phone. Comparing prices on a regular basis helps monitor and control supply costs. At least every six months, review the prices charged by different vendors for a set of frequently used items, or check several sources when a specialty item is needed. Another avenue for supply cost savings is to join one of the many medical supply discount pricing companies to receive reduced pricing on medical supplies. Most hospitals are associated with a discount buying organization and can include physician practices as part of their group. Specific group buying organizations for medical offices also exist.

Durable medical equipment supplies such as orthotics or crutches are often stocked in physicians' office for patient convenience. Reimbursement should be fully explored prior to offering this service. In addition, supplies can expire or deteriorate, so rotating stock is required. Any packaging that is yellowing or has a less-than-perfect appearance should be discarded.

Organizing supplies for ease of use can take some thought to establish, but the effort will be much appreciated by clinicians when the supply is needed.

EQUIPMENT MANAGEMENT

In any clinic, medical equipment is prevalent. The exam room, for example, contains an examination table, physician stool, blood pressure cuff (sphygmomanometer), thermometer, otoscope, ophthalmoscope, and so forth. A specialty exam room may feature a Mayo instrument stand, an electrocardiogram machine, a hyfecator, a surgical exam table, a colonoscope, and so forth. Most of these pieces also require supplies of their own and/or maintenance of some sort. Preventive maintenance should be scheduled on a regular basis to take care of this equipment. Toward this end, a maintenance checklist such as the one in **Exhibit 8.4** can be developed and updated to ensure that all the products are checked or other tasks are performed regularly.

FORMS

If the practice does not have an EMR, nursing staff may be responsible for a variety of forms related to patient visits, including progress notes, medication sheets for chart preparation, or release forms. Storing these forms in a way that allows access can be difficult, but it is key to efficiency and accuracy. Often, nursing staff stock their own drawers with forms so they can easily find them, which leads to duplicate stocking. Establishing a central form area may reduce this duplication of effort.

PATIENT EDUCATION MATERIALS

As stated in Chapter 3 on nursing functions, patient education is one of the nurse's most important roles. It can be performed using a number of formats. For example, preprinted booklets can be purchased describing any disease, surgery, or procedure. Although costly, this format may be the best education option for a practice, but, as noted below, any material handed out should be accompanied by the nurse's teaching.

EXHIBIT 8.4 Maintenance Log

Month	Jan					Feb					Mar				
Monthly Tasks															
Clean spirometer															
Inspect first aid kits															
Order medications															
Check for outdates in samples															
Verify spill kit supplies															
Weekly Tasks															
Clean and stock rooms	M	Tu	W	Th	F	M	Tu	W	Th	F	M	Tu	W	Th	F
Clean EKG machine															
Check oxygen tank															
Clean thermometers															
Change instrument lubricant															

Most of the information a patient learns at the appointment is often forgotten because of the high volume of information given, especially when the patient is presented with a new or different diagnosis. The use of patient education materials helps reinforce the teaching provided by nursing staff. In addition to obtaining preprinted brochures and handouts, materials can be created by staff with assistance from many sources on the Internet simply by typing "patient education" into any search engine. Make sure the print is large enough and the wording is simple enough for all patients to read and understand. Pharmaceutical companies or organizations may also supply patient education materials. The American Cancer Society, for example, provides literature at little or no cost. If your practice uses an electronic medical records system, it probably includes a patient education package.

Patient literacy must also be considered when creating patient education resources. Literacy here refers both to the ability to understand health care and to being able to read and write. Depending upon your patient population, you may want to research managing literacy needs of your patients more extensively.

In summary, management of clinical supplies may not be a high priority for nursing staff in the practice, but it does require some attention on the part of the clinical staff and management.

Chapter 9

Documentation

Nursing documentation in a physician's office is much different from hospital nursing documentation. Physicians may want to place restrictions on nursing documentation or, in some cases, eliminate it and provide all documentation themselves. An old nursing adage states that if you are going to perform a task, you need to document it, so some nurses who practice in an office or a clinic setting may have to reconcile their training with the physician's wishes.

In the hospital setting, the assessment of the patient starts when the nurse walks into the patient's hospital room. Is the patient alert and awake? Is the skin pink or pale, warm or clammy, dry or damp? Is the patient talking, sitting up, walking, or lying down? For the majority of a 24-hour day in the hospital, much nursing time is spent performing assessments on the patient. Nurses are the eyes and ears of the physician and thus can alert him or her to the changing status of the patient. The physician sees the patient for 10 to 15 minutes of that day and therefore depends on the nursing documentation to inform him or her of what has occurred with the patient in the last 24 hours.

Contrast that scenario to the medical office setting, in which the nurse most often performs only a small part of the patient assessment. For a normal office visit, the patient is coming to see the physician. The nursing staff's interaction with the patient is momentary, perhaps including only a quick and limited assessment; the physician performs his or her own detailed examination..

Agreement between the physician and nursing staff on what needs to be documented is vital. In one primary care office, a patient has been coming to see the physician every two months for the last two years for follow-up on his diabetes. When the nurse rooms the patient for the physician, takes his vital signs, and asks him questions, she notices the patient's appears less alert than during the previous visit. Depending on the physician's preference for documentation, the nurse might document that assessment in the chart or tell the physician of her findings. If the assessment is provided to the physician verbally, it is not particularly necessary for the nurse to document her findings, knowing the physician will do so.

If the patient is only seeing the nurse for an injection, chemotherapy, or a pro-thrombin time test, the documentation needed may require a more in-depth assessment. Flow sheets documenting the procedure are easy for the physician to review.

Nursing education places tremendous emphasis on assessment documentation. The old rule, "If it isn't documented, it wasn't done," can be heard at least a thousand times throughout nursing school. So by the time nurses graduate it has been drilled into their heads: document, document, document. In fact, it becomes quite a struggle for nurses to learn not to document.

This chapter proposes some guidelines regarding physician office documentation. First, an overview of how to perform documentation and who should document is given. Next, requirements for office visit, phone call, procedure, medication documentation, and physician orders are examined. Examples of specific documentation are included. The information provided here applies to both electronic and non-electronic formats since there is a combination of EMR and non-EMR based practices. This discussion is a brief introduction to the topic; detailed information on physician office documentation could fill volumes.

DOCUMENTATION OVERVIEW

Simple documentation dos and don'ts are described below.

Do's

- Always make sure you have the right medical record before documenting.
- Use the right ink color. Although it might be stylish to use that purple pen, it should not be used in a medical record. Black ink is preferred.
- Include the date and time for all entries. EMRs are great at doing this for you.

- Sign all entries made in the chart. For EMRs, make sure you only document when you are signed in and not on someone else's login.

- Strike through errors with one line and initial the marking. The old way to correct errors was to write "error" on top of the incorrect item. That procedure is no longer necessary. Errors show correction in an EMR. Ensure there is a policy on how to correct electronic errors.

- Document facts only (e.g., if you walk into an exam room and the patient is on the floor, document as "patient found on floor beside exam table," not that "patient fell off exam table").

- Identify late entries by labeling them as such (e.g., "late entry—patient stated he was allergic to eggs").

- Use only appropriate and standard abbreviations. If in doubt, do not abbreviate.

DON'TS

- Don't use correction fluid or obliterate mistakes; instead, cross through the entry with one line and initial.

- Don't chart for others. If an entry needs to be made for someone else, mention his or her name or position in the entry (e.g., "receptionist states he has attempted to contact patient three times to make return appointment").

- Don't express opinions (e.g., "injection given by mistake").

- Don't leave large blank spots in the chart. Each entry should directly follow the previous entry, or a line should be used to mark through empty spaces.

- Don't cover any part of the medical record. If you need to replace dictation, make a line through the wrong dictation and place the corrected dictation at the end.

WHO SHOULD DOCUMENT

Disagreement as to who should document may arise in the practice. In some specialist offices, physicians may have the receptionist notate the chief complaint in the medical record after checking the patient in for the visit. The argument is that it saves nursing staff time getting the patient in the room. However, problems can arise when front desk receptionists quiz patients regarding their office visit. In one practice, a physician wanted the reason for the visit documented in the medical record to match the appointment schedule's documentation. He was concerned that the nurse assigned to him was too busy and was forgetting to document the reason in the record. However, if the appointment schedule is not correct, then the medical record must be corrected anyway.

In this case, the appropriate way to handle documenting the reason for the visit is for the receptionist to stamp or write the date in the medical record and for nursing staff to document the reason for the visit. This physician's office solved its problem by placing a brightly colored sticky note with the reason for the visit on the progress note to remind the nurse to document the reason. Occasionally, the nurse would still forget to document, but the sticky note provided the physician with the reason for the visit. At the end of the office visit shift, the nurse would double-check all the charts, document those items she had forgotten to enter initially, and remove the sticky notes.

EXHIBIT 9.1 Communication Sheet

Room #_____ Patient name_____	Date_____
Nursing: Reason for visit _____ Wt_____ Ht____ T____ P____ BP____ R____ LMP_____ Pulse ox_____ Injury: Y N Work Comp: Y N	Doctor's assessment:
Doctor's orders Lab: CBC CMP Lipid T4 TSH PSA UA Other:_____ STAT ASAP before next visit X-ray:_____ Consult:_____ Other orders:	Return appt_____ Reason_____ _____ Rx_____ Samples_____

Some practices have the nursing assistant place the patient in the room and then have the nurse follow in to document the reason for the visit or to do the assessment. This approach was seen in a practice that used an electronic medical record (EMR). Practice administration expected a nursing assessment to be done on each patient and recorded in the EMR prior to the physician entering the room. Several physician did not want the nursing staff to document anything in the record. The solution was to introduce a colored paper communication sheet filled out by nursing that gave the physician all the pertinent information (e.g., vital signs, reason for the visit) and allowed the physician to communicate back orders and conduct her assessment (**Exhibit 9.1**). This communication sheet did not become part of the record The physician dictated details from the sheet into the EMR, and the sheet was then shredded .The important point regarding who should document is to achieve agreement on what documentation should be done prior to the physician visit.

ITEMS TO INCLUDE IN DOCUMENTATION

Different situations require different documentation. This section reviews patient visit, phone call, procedure, medication, and physician order documentation requirements.

Patient Visit Documentation

Standard visit documentation may include date, time (as appropriate), vital signs, weight, height, reason for the visit, complaints, and/or need for prescription refills (if any), and signature of nursing staff. (In some specialties, physicians may or may not require vital signs be taken.) A stamp or preprinted progress note for each visit can be used to enter these items if an EMR is not used.

Other visit documentation may include disease-specific forms. The diabetic, for example, might require a flow sheet for frequently asked questions, such as the one shown in **Exhibit 9.2, t**o be created to ensure the patient is fully assessed.[1] Flowsheets are often seen in EMRs.

This type of flow sheet can be tailored for many chronic diseases—diabetes, chronic obstructive pulmonary disease, congestive heart failure, and so forth—so that documentation can easily be reviewed and compared from year to year or visit to visit. Since many patients have comorbidities, a chronic disease flow sheet may be more useful to collect all pertinent information.

---

[1]   Kentucky Diabetes Network, Inc. 2007. "Diabetes Care Tool." www.kentuckydiabetes.net/ pdf%20files/KDN_DM_Care_Tool_7-07.pdf. (Accessed 10/15/08.)

EXHIBIT 9.2 Diabetes Care Tool

Patient Name _____ DOB _____
Height _____ Smoker Yes No (circle one)
Pneumococcal Vaccine Dates(s)_____
Type of Diabetes: 1 2 (circle one)   Year of Diagnosis_____

	Date of Visit				
Every Visit					
Weight					
B/P (goal <130/80 mmHG)					
A1C Hemoglobin A1C q 3-6 months (goal <7%)					
Annual					
Foot exam - visual					
Foot exam - Sensation, foot structure/biomechanics, vascular and skin integrity					
Fasting lipid profile - Total cholesterol (goal <200 mg/dL) - LDL (goal < 100 mg/dL) - HDL (goal men >40mg/dL, women >50 mg/dL) - Triglycerides (goal <150 mg/dL)					
Microalbumin: unless urine dipstick positive for protein					
Dilated eye exam/referral date					
Flu vaccine					
Oral visualization					
Counseling					
Self-management education/referral date					
Exercise/physical activity					
Medical nutrition therapy referral					
Tobacco cessation					
Preconception counseling (women of childbearing age)					
Other					
Review self-monitoring blood glucose log					
Assess need for aspirin therapy					

Source: Adapted with permission from the Kentucky Diabetes Network, Inc www.kentuckydiabetes.net

Similarly, flow sheets for vital signs/weight/height or child growth can be used to provide a quick graphic image for the physician to monitor health over the course of several months or years. This usage varies by practice and may include preventive health information. One practice used a checklist at the beginning of the medical record to double-check preventive care completion for each patient (**Exhibit 9.3**). This has been used also in EMRs.

EXHIBIT 9.3 Prevention Flow Sheet					
Patient name _____ DOB_____					
Service	2008	2009	2010	2011	2012
Mammogram					
Colonoscopy					
Stool hemoccult					
Pneumovax vaccine					
Influenza vaccine					
Pap smear					
Digital rectal exam					
PSA					
Lipid screening					

PHONE CALL DOCUMENTATION

Many variations exist in documentation procedures for telephone calls. Phone notes can be typed freeform or in a template. If phone calls are infrequent, then their documentation may be typed into the medical record by the nurse. If phone calls are frequent, then a template or form may be used by the reception staff to begin documentation. Instead of duplicating the receptionist's efforts, the nurse documents his or her assessment and actions below the phone call note. An example of a paper template that can be transposed into an EMR for a phone note is shown in **Exhibit 9.4**.

The phone note may include the following:

- Date and time of call;
- Patient name, date of birth;

- Who made the call;
- Phone number(s) and availability;
- Physician involved;
- Reason for call;
- If symptom call, list of symptoms, duration, treatments tried;
- If medication refill, medication, dosage, frequency, name of pharmacy, pharmacy number, urgency of refill, date of last refill;
- Medication allergies; and
- Space for follow-up on nursing actions, physician orders.

EXHIBIT 9.4 Phone Note					
Dr 1 2 3 4 5 6 7 8	Date and time:	Patient name and DOB:			
__allergies __chest pain __ cough - prod __congestion __diarrhea __dizziness __fatigue __fever	__headache __nasal drainage __ nausea __pain __rash __sore throat __short of breath __vomiting				
		Patient phone #	Pharmacy and phone #	Allergies	
Physician orders/nursing care given:					

For practices with EMR, documentation is much simplified. A phone call note template can be set up in the EMR that greatly streamlines the nurse's documentation process.

PROCEDURE DOCUMENTATION

When nursing staff perform a procedure without the assistance of the physician (e.g., dressing change, application of cast, irrigation of catheter, ear lavage), nursing should document that procedure. Nursing may also document continuous assessments before, during, or after procedures performed by the physician (e.g., cardiac testing, colonoscopy). Documentation should include:

- Date and time;

- Specific measures taken;

- Assessment of the patient (e.g., wound, findings during the procedure); and

- Follow-up, if indicated.

Usually, free-form notes are used to document nursing procedures. However, flow sheets may facilitate continuous documentation (**Exhibit 9.5**).

EXHIBIT 9.5 Procedure Flow Sheet					
Date_____ Patient name_____					
Time	Pulse	Respiration	BP Sitting	BP Lying	Nursing Documentation

Prothrombin time (protime) clinic visits or blood pressure checks can be documented on a form specifically designed for that clinic and incorporated into the EMR (**Exhibit 9.6**).

EXHIBIT 9.6 Flow Sheet

Patient name_____
Diagnosis_____ Physician_____

Date	INR	Protime	Current Dosage	Change in Dosage	Patient Notified

One necessary type of documentation is the consent to treatment form. Written consents should be obtained for any procedure performed in the office. Some procedures fall within a gray area in determining whether they need consent. If the physician sees the patient, diagnoses a broken arm, and tells the patient the nurse will apply a cast, the physician has documented agreement with the treatment option in his note. Thus, a consent is probably not needed. However, if the physician sees the patient, examines a suspicious lesion, and tells the patient he will remove the lesion, consent is probably needed. Many different types of consent exist, but the basic items for any consent form should include:

- Date;
- Physician who is performing the procedure;
- Patient's name;
- Description of the procedure;
- Explanation of the procedure and/or that an explanation has been given;
- Understanding of the risks, hazards, and outcomes of the procedure;
- Opportunity provided to the patient to ask questions;
- Agreement that no guarantee has been offered as to the results of the procedure;

- Understanding that the physician may need to perform other procedures depending on the circumstances and his or her judgment;

- Consent to anesthetics, including local;

- Consent to allow study or disposal of the tissue that is removed, if needed;

- Signature by the patient or other authorized person; and

- Signature by a witness.

A lawyer should be consulted when drafting a consent form to ensure that all of the necessary components are included. An example of a minor surgery consent form is displayed in **Exhibit 9.7**.

EXHIBIT 9.7 Minor Procedure Consent Form

Minor Procedure Consent

I, _____ , consent to

Dr. _____ performing the following procedure:

_____

_____

_____

The procedure and risks associated with the procedure have been explained to me, and I have had the opportunity to ask questions. Because I will be awake during the procedure, the physician may discuss other procedures he or she feels are necessary during the course of this procedure.

I also consent to the administration of local anesthetics.

_____

Signature of patient

_____

Witness

MEDICATION DOCUMENTATION

Administration of medication should always be documented by the nurse who gives the medication. Documentation should include medication, dose, route, time and date, patient's response to the medication, and instructions given to the patient allowing for adequate follow-up.

Documentation of medication administration varies from practice to practice. For an oncology office, a flow sheet with chemotherapy administration may be used in conjunction with a medication log for injections. An allergy office may have a separate injection log for allergy shot administration. Often, injections given in a primary care office will be documented in the medication record of the EMR. An example of an allergy injection flow sheet is shown in **Exhibit 9.8**.

EXHIBIT 9.8 Allergy Injection Treatment Record

Patient Name _____   DOB _____

Date	Antigen	Dil.	Vial/ amt.	Arm	Reaction/Tx	Remarks	Initials
				R L			
				R L			
				R L			
				R L			
				R L			
				R L			
				R L			
				R L			
				R L			
				R L			

PHYSICIAN ORDER DOCUMENTATION

Documentation of physician orders is required for facility admissions (hospital or nursing home), community resources (home health, durable medical equipment), testing (lab or radiology), and medications.

Standing orders are useful for arranging surgery orders, hospital admissions, and nursing home admissions. If needed, the facility can provide an example of other physician orders to help develop the standing order. Once the standing order is in place, the nursing staff can pull the order for that particular diagnosis or surgery, individualize it to the patient's needs, obtain the physician's signature, and fax it to the hospital or facility.

In summary, documentation in a medical office is different from that in a hospital, but similar dos and don'ts apply. Clarification of documentation with the providers can ensure appropriate documentation is performed by all.

Chapter 10

Regulations

Numerous regulations affect clinical practice in a medical office, including those mandated by the nurse practice act of the state in which the practice operates, the Occupational Safety and Health Administration (OSHA), the Health Insurance Portability and Accountability Act (HIPAA), and the Centers for Disease Control and Prevention (CDC). Clinical trial regulations are covered at the end of the chapter. This discussion does not explore the complete list of regulations but rather highlights the chief rules that apply specifically to clinical practices.

NURSE PRACTICE ACTS

State nurse practice acts regulate the licensure and practice of nursing and provide nursing definitions for the state. Refer to Chapter 2 for a more detailed discussion of these acts and their regulations. A state's medical bylaws may also regulate nursing functions supervised by physicians. Be sure to check with your state on who supervises medical assistants.

OCCUPATIONAL SAFETY AND HEALTH ADMINISTRATION

OSHA's rules seem complicated and imposing to most people, but if procedures are developed to administer the regulations correctly, compliance can be simplified. Contrary to some beliefs, OSHA inspections do occur in medical offices. (**Exhibit 10.1**). Making some basic preparations and establishing procedures can ensure that the practice will be found in compliance if OSHA should inspect it. OSHA's website, www.osha.gov is a great resource for developing your procedures. It includes sample procedures that need only minor customization for the practice. It can also helperify that your office is conducting its operations in accordance with OSHA regulations.

EXHIBIT 10.1 OSHA Inspections

Type of Clinic	Sept. 2003-Sept. 2004	Sept. 2004-Sept. 2005	Sept. 2005-Sept. 2006	Sept. 2006-Sept. 2007	Sept. 2007-Sept. 2008
SIC 801 Offices and clinics of medical doctors	296	299	269	346	247
SIC 803 Offices of osteopathic physicians	6	1	1	5	1
SIC 809 Health and allied services not elsewhere classified	451				

Often, a practice carries out OSHA compliance based on a staff member's memory of the procedures learned at another facility, such as a hospital setting. Reading the regulation itself gives clear guidance to ensure proper compliance. Misinterpretation and over-interpretation are common miscues in attempts at OSHA compliance.

It is not uncommon to hear office staff misquote OSHA's requirements as being more inclusive than they actually are. One example is wearing sandals in the work setting. In one of OSHA's standard interpretation statements, a question is posed asking whether OSHA requires employees to wear shoes and socks. OSHA's response is that the employer is responsible for ensuring the employee is protected. If a reasonable chance exists that the employee will be exposed to blood and body fluids, the employer is responsible for providing shoe covers (engineering controls). However, the employer may also establish their own standards for what employees should wear, and enforce it—standards that have nothing to do with OSHA regulations.[1] OSHA does not state that wearing sandals is not allowed; but the practice's safety policy may state shoe protocol.

The aim of this section is to help the practice assess its current OSHA compliance procedures or help it establish an OSHA procedure if none exists. As it pertains to the clinical portion of the practice, OSHA is made up of two standards:

1. Bloodborne pathogen standard

2. Hazardous communication standard

Several topics that fall under OSHA's purview do not have specific standards; however, some guidance is given for the following areas:

- Tuberculosis (TB)
- Ergonomics
- General duty clause

OSHA compliance procedure implementation should be included as part of an overall general safety statement developed by the practice. OSHA regulation adherence constitutes only one portion of overall safety in your practice.

OSHA requires the practice to inform employees of their exposure to potential health hazards related to their job and to make sure employees are working in a safe environment. This requirement includes the following:

- Training upon employment and every year thereafter. Specific training requirements are written in each standard.

- A safety officer on staff to provide direction in safety issues.

- Record-keeping, including attendance records for training programs and maintenance of occupational exposure records.

The rest of this section summarizes OSHA requirements.

---

[1]   Occupational Safety and Health Administration, U.S. Department of Labor. 2006. "Wearing Sandals in a Medical Office when Feet Do Not Contact Blood or OPIM." www.osha.gov/pls/oshaweb/owadisp.show_document?p_table=INTERPRETATIONS&p_id=25497. (Accessed 9/1/08.)

BLOODBORNE PATHOGENS STANDARD 29 CFR 1910.1030

This standard was created to help prevent or reduce exposures to bloodborne pathogens.

- Exposure determination. One of the first things to determine in any practice is the exposure of the employees. Every job should be listed, and a determination regarding exposure for each should be identified.

- Implementation of exposure control methods. Identifying, teaching, and using the following controls are required:

  Hand washing.

  Personal protective equipment. This includes gloves, gowns, and masks. In 2001, this portion was revised with the addition of the Needlestick Safety and Prevention Act, which requires the review and implementation of needleless devices.

  Housekeeping. Disposal of sharps and regulated waste and a written schedule of cleaning and laundry are covered in this section.

- Hepatitis B vaccination. Using the exposure determination, those employees exposed to blood should be offered the vaccination free of charge within 10 days of assignment to those areas. If the employee declines the vaccination, he or she should sign a declination form.

- Post-exposure evaluation. If an employee is exposed to blood, a defined procedure should be in place to follow.

- Training. Training should be given upon hire and annually.

- Record-keeping:

  Training. Specific requirements mandate recording of training.

  Hepatitis B injection.

   Exposure medical records. These records should not be part of the regular medical chart. They should be kept in a separate file.

  Sharps injury log. Specific requirements mandate recording, and the log should be reviewed annually.[2]

---

[2]   Occupational Safety and Health Administration, U.S. Department of Labor. 2003. "Model Plans and Programs for the OSHA Bloodborne Pathogens and Hazard Communications Standards." www.osha.gov/Publications/osha3186.html. (Accessed 9/1/08.)

HAZARDOUS COMMUNICATION STANDARD 29 CFR 1910.1200

This standard is meant to inform employees of the hazardous chemicals with which they work, safe handling procedures, and protection measures from these hazards. It includes the following:

- Hazard determination and list of hazardous chemicals. If specific hazardous chemicals are involved in a task, they should be identified. All chemicals that are used in the practice should be listed.

- Material Safety Data Sheet (MSDS). All chemicals require an MSDS that is easily accessible in case an employee has been exposed to that chemical.

- Container labeling. Specific requirements dictate how to label containers.

- Storage and handling of hazardous chemicals. Specific requirements mandate where and how these chemicals can be stored.

- Chemical spills. A procedure should be identified for such an occurrence, including the availability of eyewash stations.

- Training. Specific requirements regulate training at initial hire and review as necessary.

TUBERCULOSIS AND RESPIRATORY PROTECTION

OSHA refers to the CDC's .Guidelines for Preventing the Transmission of Mycobacterium tuberculosis in Health-Care Settings, 2005 for guidance on TB[3]. The new Guidelines state that all healthcare settings need a TB infection control program which is based on administrative, environmental and respiratory protection. An overview of the recommendations for a medical office are the following:

- Administrative controls to reduce the risk for exposure to persons who might have TB disease,

- Assigning responsibility for TB infection control;

- Conducting a TB risk assessment;

- Developing and instituting a written TB infection-control plan;

---

3   CDC, Guidelines for Preventing the Transmission of Mycobacterium tuberculosis in Health-Care Settings, 2005, http://www.cdc.gov/mmwr/preview/mmwrhtml/rr5417a1.htm?s_cid=rr5417a1_e (accessed 3.3.2016)

- Implementing effective work practices for the management of patients with suspected or confirmed TB disease;

- Training and educating health care workers regarding TB, with specific focus on prevention, transmission, and symptoms;

- Screening and evaluating health care workers who are at risk for TB disease or who might be exposed to M. tuberculosis;

- Using appropriate signage advising respiratory hygiene and cough etiquette; and

- Coordinating efforts with the local or state health department.

- Guidance on when infected employees can return to work.

- Environmental Controls to prevent the spread and reduce the concentration of the infectious droplets such ventilation and appropriate HEPA filters.

- Respiratory Protection Controls for those patients with infectious TB disease such as implementing a respiratory protection program, training health care workers on respiratory protection and training patients on respiratory hygiene and cough etiquette.

ERGONOMICS GUIDANCE

OSHA has issued guidelines to some industries for reducing musculoskeletal injuries in the workplace. In health care, only guidelines for the nursing home industry have been released. OSHA is encouraging other industries to develop ergonomic guidance for their workplace-specific needs.

Some practices bring in an occupational therapist to review work practices and to offer suggestions on reducing potential risks for injuries. Areas of concern may include height of the chair in relation to the desk, proper use of the computer to reduce back and neck pain, and lifting mechanics.

GENERAL DUTY CLAUSE

Any safety measure not covered in the above regulations and guidelines may fall under the general duty clause of OSHA, which states that:

• Employers shall furnish employees a place free from recognized hazards that are causing death or physical harm to employees;

• Employers shall comply with the OSHA standards; and

- Employees shall comply with OSHA rules, regulations, and orders issued.[4]

Under this clause, a practice should implement escape procedures and routes in case of emergency (e.g., disaster, fire, tornado, earthquake). It should include a means of accounting for all individuals and a means of reporting emergencies. In the course of this implementation, the practice may also address hallway clearance, electrical safety, and similar concerns.

Recordkeeping

Employers with 10 employees or fewer in certain industry classifications are partially exempt from keeping injury and illness records. This exemption may pertain to your practice, but in the health care industry, numerous hazards occur, behooving you to follow OSHA guidelines. This author's recommendation is that all medical practices have OSHA regulation procedures in place.

In addition, certain OSHA Standard Industrial Classification codes do not require filing an OSHA 200 log (codes are given in parentheses):

- Offices and clinics of medical doctors (801)
- Offices and clinics of dentists (802)
- Offices of osteopathic physicians (803)
- Medical and dental laboratories (807)
- Health and allied services not elsewhere classified (809)

All employers must report to OSHA any workplace incident that results in a death or the hospitalization of three or more employees in specific time frames, providing specific information about the incidents. Reportable incidents include a heart attack experienced by someone while at work. Once reported, OSHA decides whether to investigate the incident for possible violations.

HEALTH INSURANCE PORTABILITY AND ACCOUNTABILITY ACT

The Health Information Portability and Accountability Act (HIPAA) of 1996 includes guidelines for clinical staff regarding the privacy and security of protected health information. As health care providers, all nursing staff are covered under the act. Protected health information is that with which clinical staff work daily in electronic, paper, and oral form.

---

4   Occupational Safety and Health Administration, U.S. Department of Labor. 1970. OSHA Act of 1970. www.osha.gov/pls/oshaweb/owadisp.show_document?p_table=OSHACT&p_id=3359. (Accessed 9/1/08.)

One of the main concerns of HIPAA for clinical staff is the treatment of patients. The clinical staff, a covered entity, can use and disclose protected health information for treatment, payment, and health care operations without obtaining consent from the patient. Following HIPAA guidelines can become tricky when working with other health care providers. Most often, few problems arise when releasing information if the patient is referred to another provider. However, if another practice asks for records and your practice did not refer the patient to that practice, consent may be required and used as a communication tool, if nothing else.

Some hospitals enforce HIPAA beyond the treatment option. For example, a surgical practice may not be able to obtain radiology films from the screening facility on the patient's behalf without the patient's consent. HIPAA's guidelines on privacy can be interpreted in many ways, and nursing staff may need to clarify those issues that relate to their practice.

Once they give consent, patients can change their mind regarding whether they want records transferred. One occurrence at a physician's practice brought this eventuality home: A patient signed a consent form at a research facility for the facility to obtain all records from a medical office. After leaving the research facility, the patient changed his mind and decided that he did not want to participate in the research study. He called the practice and insisted his records not be released. In the event such a situation occurs in your practice, make sure a system is in place for patients to retract any previously given consent.

It is important for nursing staff to understand how HIPAA affects them in day-to-day situations. For instance, if they are treating a patient who is accompanied by a police officer, how much can the staff tell the police officer? Who can they talk to about a specific patient? Can a divorced father not living with a child-patient be told of his child's condition?

Instructions to nursing staff on how to handle custody issues with divorced parents help nursing navigate some very touchy conversations. The same holds true for foster care arrangements and family members of incarcerated patients. At one clinic, the mother of a man who was in prison called to find out the time of her son's doctor's appointment. The receptionist, not aware that the patient was in custody, gave out the appointment time. The family showed up at the clinic to see the prisoner on an unsupervised visit. Giving nursing staff and the receptionist guidance can help them head off any issues that may arise. Simple discussions of tricky situations can also help ensure that the right actions will result when the nursing staff are faced with a difficult situation.

The list of designated individuals who have access to patient information can be placed in the practice management software, electronic medical record, or medical chart so the nursing staff can determine immediately if they are permitted to talk with the inquiring person.

A key concept for clinical staff to adhere to is "minimum necessary": Staff should obtain or send only that information necessary to treat the patient.

Accounting for disclosures may cause difficulty as well. Clinicians copy and send records to various other clinicians involved in the care of the patient. To keep track of these disclosures, make sure a note in the chart indicates where the records have been sent.

Patient confidentiality issues can arise in many forms and arenas. For example, talking in the hallway about a patient or having a conversation at a restaurant about patient circumstances can lead to breach-of-privacy problems. A constant reminder to all staff is needed to ensure the utmost care is taken with communications.[5]

CENTERS FOR DISEASE CONTROL AND PREVENTION

The Centers for Disease Control and Prevention website has a wealth of knowledge to be used in the clinical setting. On matters from handwashing techniques to isolation procedures for certain diseases, the CDC has issued guidance. One of the most notorious guidelines is that regarding universal precautions. These guidelines were developed in the late 1980s in response to the HIV threat. Prior to the 1987 CDC guideline, nurses were not required to wear gloves during procedures. This guideline has changed the face of infection control like nothing else.[6,7]

Resources for the CDC, National Institute for Occupational Safety and Health (NIOSH), and OSHA are included in **Exhibit 10.2** for further review.

---

5   U.S. Department of Health and Human Services. HIPAA for Professionals, http://www.hhs.gov/hipaa/for-professionals/index.html, (accessed 3.3.2016)

6   Centers for Disease Control and Prevention.2007 Guideline for Isolation Precautions: Preventing Transmission of Infectious Agents in Healthcare Settings, http://www.cdc.gov/hicpac/2007IP/2007isolationPrecautions.html (accessed 3.3.2016)

7   Centers for Disease Control and Prevention. Recommendations for Prevention of HIV Transmission in Health-Care Settings, The National Institute for Occupational Safety and Health (NIOSH), http://www.cdc.gov/niosh/topics/bbp/universal.html (accessed 3.3.2016)

EXHIBIT 10.2 Resource Numbers	
CDC	www.cdc.gov
	Health and safety topics on numerous topics
Federal OSHA site	www.osha.gov
	Compliance assistance
	e-tools (PowerPoint presentations)
	posters
	quick cards
	Regulations
	Safety and health topics
	biological agents (bloodborne pathogens)
	emergency preparedness
	ergonomics
	hazard communications
NIOSH	www.cdc.gov/niosh/
	Health and safety guidelines on numerous topics
OSHA site index	www.osha.gov/html/a-z-index.html
To report a fatality	1.800.321.OSHA

CLINICAL TRIALS

Nursing is a key element in the implementation of a clinical trial. As implementation gets under way, the study coordinator should be available to explain and answer questions regarding protocol and regulations. Following is a brief overview of clinical trials.

Clinical trials are research studies on human volunteers conducted to answer specific health care questions. The different types of clinical trials include the following:

- Treatment trials test experimental treatments, new combinations of drugs, or new approaches to medical care.

- Prevention trials seek better ways to prevent disease, including medications, vaccines, vitamins, minerals, and lifestyle changes.

- Diagnostic trials seek better tests or procedures for diagnosis of diseases.

- Screening trials aim to determine the best way to detect certain diseases.

- Quality-of-life trials explore ways to improve comfort and quality of life for those patients with chronic illnesses.[8]

Clinical trials are sponsored and funded by many organizations and individuals, including physicians, medical institutions, foundations, voluntary groups, pharmaceutical companies, and federal agencies such as the National Institutes of Health, the Department of Defense, and the Department of Veterans Affairs.

Clinical drug trials are conducted in phases, and each phase has a different purpose to help answer different research questions.

- *Phase I.* A small group of people is tested first to evaluate safety, identify safe dosage range, and determine any side effects of drug in question. This group usually is composed of healthy volunteers. The emphasis of this phase is on safety.

- *Phase II.* A larger group of people is used to evaluate drug effectiveness and to further evaluate safety. This phase aims to obtain preliminary data on how the drug works on certain diseases or conditions. For controlled trials, patients may receive the drug being studied, a placebo (an inactive substance), or a different drug. The emphasis is on effectiveness.

- *Phase III.* In this phase, a large group of people is tested to confirm effectiveness, monitor side effects, compare the drug to commonly used treatments, and further evaluate safety issues.

- *Phase IV.* Additional information is obtained in this phase on the drug's risks, benefits, and optimal use.[9]

- In drug trials, the phases of clinical trials begin after the sponsor of the drug provides the U.S. Food and Drug Administration (FDA) with results of preclinical testing conducted on laboratory animals and indicates how it proposes to conduct testing on humans. The FDA then decides whether it is safe to proceed with testing.[10]

---

8   National Institutes of Health. 2007. "Understanding Clinical Trials." www.clinicaltrials.gov/ct2/info/understand. (Accessed 11/15/08 & 3.3.2016.)

9   National Institutes of Health. 2007. "Understanding Clinical Trials." www.clinicaltrials.gov/ct2/info/understand. (Accessed 11/15/08 & 3.3.2016.), U.S. Food and Drug Administration. n.d. "The FDA's Drug Review Process: Ensuring Drugs Are Safe and Effective."

10   U.S. Food and Drug Administration. n.d. "The FDA's Drug Review Process: Ensuring Drugs Are Safe and Effective http://www.fda.gov/drugs/resourcesforyou/consumers/ucm143534.htm (accessed 3.3.2016)

Phase IV studies are conducted after the FDA approves the drug for marketing. To obtain this approval, the drug sponsor submits a New Drug Application to the FDA. It includes all the details of the phase I–III testing as well as analysis of the data. The FDA has 60 days to approve the filing; upon approval, the drug is reviewed. The review process occurs no later than 10 months after the review has begun on 90 percent of drugs. For priority drugs, the review process goal is six months. Accelerated approval is given to those drugs meant to treat serious or life-threatening illnesses that currently lack satisfactory treatments (e.g., HIV drugs). These drugs continue to undergo studies after they are on the market and can be withdrawn if the studies do not confirm the initial results. The FDA continues to track approved drugs for adverse events and safety for two years, or three years for potentially dangerous drugs. It is during this initial period that identification of adverse side effects often occur and the FDA acts by withdrawing or limiting the drug's use.U.S. Food and Drug Administration. Every clinical trial is approved by and monitored through an institutional review board (IRB). The IRB ensures that the study is ethical and safe. It establishes and monitors the protocol, which describes the patients participating, schedule of tests, procedures, medications and dosages, and length of the study.

Inclusion and exclusion criteria for the trial are established to allow or disallow participants in the study. The criteria are based on age, gender, type and stage of the disease, previous treatment history, and other medical conditions. The informed consent process enables the patient to learn about the study: its purpose, duration, required procedures, key contacts, risks, and potential benefits.[11]

Payment or compensation may be provided to the participants and/or the physician acting as administrator of the trial. A potential conflict of interest may result if the provider is obtaining reimbursement to enroll patients in the study. This information may or may not be discussed during the informed consent process, but an informed patient may feel free to ask about reimbursement and any conflicts.

Oncology practices can benefit from the countless research studies conducted on how to treat cancers. Both patients and clinical staff can research clinical study options on many websites, including clinicaltrials.gov, a service of the National Institutes of Health.[12]

---

11   National Institutes of Health. 2007. "Understanding Clinical Trials." www.clinicaltrials.gov/ct2/info/understand. (Accessed 11/15/08 & 3.3.2016.)

12   U.S. Food and Drug Administration. n.d. "Basic Questions and Answers about Clinical Trials." http://www.fda.gov/ForConsumers/ucm121345.htm (accessed 3.3.2016).

In addition to the FDA, other agencies offer guidelines for safe clinical studies, including E6 Good Clinical Practice: Consolidated Guidance, copublished by the U.S. Department of Health and Human Services, the FDA, the Center for Drug Evaluation and Research, and the Center for Biologics Evaluation and Research. This document provides the "ethical and scientific quality standard for designing, conducting, recording, and reporting trials that involve the participation of human subjects."[13] The World Health Organization has also published guidance in this area in its "Guidelines for Good Clinical Practice (GCP) for Trials on Pharmaceutical Products." This report provides a "set of globally applicable standards for the conduct of such biomedical research on human subjects."[14] Both of these documents define and clarify expectations for clinical trials.

In summary, although additional regulations affect nursing, those mentioned in this chapter are critical for nursing staff to understand, as they directly affect their practice.

---

[13]　　Center for Drug Evaluation and Research, U.S. Food and Drug Administration. 1996. Guidance for Industry—E6 Good Clinical Practice: Consolidated Guidance.

[14]　　World Health Organization. 1995. "Guidelines for Good Clinical Practice (GCP) for Trials on Pharmaceutical Products." www.who.int/medicinedocs/collect/medicinedocs/pdf/whozip13e/whozip13e.pdf. (Accessed 11/15/08 & 3.3.2016.)

Chapter 11

Other Management Issues

There is so much more to the management of the clinical area of the medical practice than those points discussed in the previous chapters. In addition to the foregoing, clinical management has the added complexity of intimately involving the physician in the day-to-day operations. This chapter examines some unique challenges of managing the nursing department.

NURSING CAREER

Nursing is a tough career, especially for the uninitiated. Experienced nurses tend to guard the territory and "eat their young." These nurses, consciously or not, tend to place roadblocks in the way of young nurses, testing them and potentially impeding their success. There is nothing as frightful for a new nurse as taking on that first patient without the teacher standing behind him or her. On the other hand, there is nothing more exhilarating than saving a life or being involved in a crisis that turns out well. Living through a crisis that does not turn out well is also part of learning. If a new nurse does the right things and remains cool, he becomes "one of us." If he fails, he has to try again.

To an experienced nurse on the hospital floor, the administration can also be the enemy. All clinical activities happen outside administration's realm, perpetuating an "administration does not understand" mentality. An "entry fee" into the field is required, which may be difficult for a graduate nurse to figure out and even more difficult for a non-clinician to determine.

Today, preceptor programs ease these burdens on the new nurse. Nursing leaders understand that new nurses are needed to sustain the profession, and they have tried to ease the transition from student to practicing nurse. Hospital administration is supporting this effort.

MEDICAL PRACTICE MENTALITY

The nursing mentality of the medical practice is very different from that of the hospital. In the hospital, nursing finds itself in the middle between physician and hospital. Nurses, as employees of the hospital, must comply with the hospital's rules to remain employed. At the same time, they have to work with the physicians, who are often at odds with administration, to take care of the patients.

In a medical practice, the physician most often rules, and patient care becomes the primary objective. Bureaucracy is minimal, fewer policies and procedures are in place in the office than in the hospital, and initiatives are implemented only to improve patient care. The mentality is patient care friendly, which pleases both physicians and nursing.

If something or someone hinders the ability of either the physician or the nurse to care for their patients, an "us versus them" mind-set can result. Administration has to understand this concept, because nurses and physicians may stand together against administration if they feel threatened.

NURSE AS A CAREGIVER

Often encountered in medical practices are those nurses who want to just do nursing. In hospitals, nursing's primary role is patient care. Other departments are created to handle all the "other stuff" related to the patient's stay, such as insurance, coding, billing, discharge planning, social work, and infection control—the hospital nurse cares little about how the bill is paid.

In most medical practices, however, other tasks often require nursing's attention. Nursing has to understand the dynamics of coding, billing, and insurance in order for the practice to be successful. Nursing staff must deal with a multitude of variables related to community resources, durable medical equipment, home health, referrals, and pharmaceutical companies. Practicing in a physician's office is a huge change for a nurse transitioning from the hospital setting. In this situation, nurses need training specific to the practice because they are on the front line dealing with these issues.

To avoid providing such training, some managers may decide to hire only nurses who do not have hospital experience. But this is a flawed approach, as hospital experience is necessary to the development of a good office nurse.

NURSE-PHYSICIAN RELATIONSHIP

As the nurse-physician relationship lengthens, the two parties become more at-tuned to each other's likes and dislikes. Multiple day-to-day decisions are made that are critical in the care of the patient. The physician and nurse start to depend on each other, and the relationship solidifies. The trust between the two deepens. In a good working relationship, the nurse may anticipate the physician's needs before the physician recognizes them. For example, nurses who have an aligned relationship with the physician know the physician's preferences for how his or her day should run. Perhaps a scheduling issue has occurred that the nurse expects will upset the physician. The nurse acts by adjusting patients' appoint-ments to reduce the possibility of ruining the physician's day. This attention is good for the practice, as it results in happy doctors.

Unfortunately, this relationship can overlap into other parts of their lives. It is not uncommon for one physician to have his nurse ask the drug representative for extra samples for his wife's condition or for another to prevail upon the nurse to watch her children so that she and her husband can go out to dinner. The nurse might spend a large sum of money on a personal holiday or birthday gifts for the physician or vice versa. Communication exhibited between the physician and nurse may be different from that between the physician and other staff. Further, the relationship may take on a different complexion than that of colleagues if these "favors" or exclusive communications continue to escalate. In that event, a professional relationship no longer exists between the two, and the employer—the manager—has been removed from the dynamic.

At times, the nurse-physician relationship may become unhealthy, problems may result between the nurse and physician, and the practice as a whole may suffer. An extension of this relationship shift is a physician and nurse having an affair with each other. Another manifestation may be the physician defending the nurse's wrongdoings so that he will not lose the relationship with the nurse. Sim-ilarly, a physician may "hurt the feelings" of the nurse, engendering empathy for the nurse from other staff. All these scenarios can disrupt the office practice.

A strong professional, caring relationship between the nurse and physician is crucial for the office to run smoothly. The physician should trust the nursing staff and provide them with autonomy to do their job. He or she should respect their role and the functions of the position. Likewise, the nursing staff should respect the physician's position. Professionalism between the two should be ev-ident—including staff refraining from using the physician's first name. Others may disagree on the necessity of this rule, but experiences has lent credence to the philosophy that physicians should be called "Doctor" by all staff. This boundary establishes and maintains that essential professional relationship. The role of the doctor and nurse should be very clear to all.

If the relationship between physician and nurse becomes more than professional, some clarification is needed for both staff and physician. The nurse is employed at the office to work at the office, not to be the physician's personal attendant. The latter situation is detrimental to the nurse and can be difficult for the practice, and it has to be addressed. Administration must step in when the first signs of crossing the line occur. Taking measures to detour such a relationship becomes much more difficult as the relationship changes and time passes. The practice's ruling board should be clear on physician-nurse relationships. Consult its standards to define the practice's policy, and enforce it.

NURSE AS THE GATEKEEPER

Nursing can readily identify with the physician in terms of carrying out processes and procedures because the focus is mostly on patient care. Thus, the nurse becomes the gatekeeper to the physician concerning calls from outside the office as well as inquiries from other staff inside the office. The nurse determines who sees and who does not see the physician. So the power that the nurse may have in any given office situation is great. Because the physician is the most powerful person in the practice and the nurse controls who has access to the physician, the nurse by extension becomes more powerful in the practice. Nursing can use this power well or use it destructively.

Nurses sometimes feel they are closer to the physician than any other person in the office, including the administrator. They can use this relationship to gain preferential treatment in decisions made by the ruling board. One example of this preferred treatment may be to lobby the physician for increased vacation time for nursing staff over that of office staff. The physician may be convinced that nursing works harder and therefore needs more time off. Or the nurse may use his or her relationship with the physician to hurt other members of the team. Quite often, the nurse has the physician's ear while others on staff have a hard time gaining access to him or her. Sometimes, the nurse is so adept and subtle in this effort that the physician does not even realize he or she is being manipulated. It is important for administration to identify the situation and clarify the nurse's role when it suspects this scenario is developing.

NURSING PERFORMANCE PROBLEMS

It is sometimes hard to determine whether a nursing performance problem exists if no one complains. Not uncommon are occasions in which a nursing staff member leaves and then everyone tells all about his or her deficiencies. Unless direct supervision of nursing is conducted—and even when it is—uncovering competency problems may be difficult. The physician knows that "something is wrong" but cannot identify the problem. Switching nursing staff from working with one physician to working with another for a week or a few days can reveal performance issues to the physicians and to others. If the practice has a clinical supervisor, having the supervisor work with a particular physician for a day or two may uncover issues just by the ensuing questions that will arise while the nurse is performing procedures. In addition, physicians should always be included in performance reviews that identify specific behaviors. Adhering to objective performance criteria is difficult for a clinician to fake. Sometimes, more training or finding a different position that better suits that person is the answer when nursing performance issues arise.

FAVORITISM

Good treatment of a well-run nursing staff by a physician is often interpreted as favoritism by non-clinical staff. Physicians may act on or give voice to their appreciation of nursing in different ways than they do with other people in the office. The physician may visit with one staff member more often than others. She may feel more comfortable with nursing staff than office staff because she understands their role. There may or may not be favoritism; the physician may just be happy that she has a well-run department. Administration needs to work with both clinical and office staff to allay any concerns about these relationship quirks or to address them if the treatment truly results in favoritism.

BAD APPLES

Sometimes a manager knows a problem exists but cannot pinpoint the exact cause. His gut tells him that a certain person is the cause and everything points in the direction of the troublemaker. Issues that arise may not be rooted in blatant breaches of policy but do trigger subtle, nagging apprehension, feeding an undercurrent of unease but pointing to nothing substantial to back up growing concerns. Examine this feeling closely to specify the nature of the issue.

As with any office environment, one employee can have a huge impact—especially one who has a bad or scheming attitude. As the adage goes, one bad apple can spoil the whole bunch. Usually, when your gut tells you something is just not right, follow your gut—get rid of bad apples. The turnaround in productivity and morale for the entire office will validate your action.

MEDICAL STUDENTS AND RESIDENTS

Medical students or residents might be frequent additions to a medical practice if the physician enjoys teaching. Most educational programs provide information about the student or resident, including his or her credentials or education level, liability carrier, and evaluation from the program. The practice should develop a protocol to ensure that these students/residents are familiar with practice procedures, including the privacy rule portion of the Health Insurance Portability and Accountability Act, patient flow, Occupational Safety and Health Administration regulations, coding, transcription, and billing. An information packet can be individualized to the practice and describe what the student/resident is allowed to do. A file of all past students/residents should be kept in case of liability concerns that may later develop.

PROBLEM PHYSICIANS

A physician who has either a problem behavior or a bad attitude can be detrimental to the functioning of the clinical department. He or she will not only require more work from the nursing staff but also affect every department. If the practice experiences problems hiring and keeping staff for a physician, delve into the situation to determine the issues at play for that particular physician. He or she may be part of the problem.

Most often, nursing and physicians work in harmony with few problems. Being aware of any potential issues, however, prepares you to address them when they arise in the office.

Chapter 12

Ancillary Services

A book on clinical management in a medical practice would not be complete without reference to ancillary services. Ancillary services can be broken down into several categories:

- Diagnostic testing
  - Lab
  - Radiology
  - Nuclear medicine
- Other modalities
  - Physical therapy
  - Occupational therapy
  - Respiratory therapy
  - Pain management
  - Cosmetic injections
- Retail
  - Pharmacy
  - Optical shops
  - Cosmetic and skin care products
  - Orthotics

Most of the ideas presented in previous chapters can be applied to ancillary services. This chapter looks briefly at each concept as it applies to the various services.

THE RIGHT STAFF

The right staff is important to any department or division. Understanding the education and licensure of those staff is necessary.

DIAGNOSTIC TESTING

The education and licensure requirements of laboratory personnel depend on the certification agency used by the lab. Numerous national certification programs exist for the various types of diagnostic allied health personnel, including those listed in **Exhibit 12.1**.

EXHIBIT 12.1 Clinical Laboratory Staffing

Medical technologist
> Schooling: 4-year degree
> National certification

Laboratory technician
> Schooling: 2-year degree
> National certification

Medical laboratory technician
> Schooling: none
> Registration: none
> Experience and testing required

Certified office laboratory technician
> Schooling: none
> Registration: none
> Experience and testing required
> Certification available

Phlebotomist
> Schooling: training on the job for up to 1 year
> Certification available

As with nursing, a more experienced staff can be instrumental in making the lab work flow efficiently. Certain regulations require the use of a medical technologist to supervise the lab staff. Of course, the more educated and experienced staff will be paid more than those with less training and experience. A phlebotomist position may be the lowest paid person in the lab, but the regulations they must know and comply with are extensive. For instance, Medicare only authorizes reimbursement on a complete blood count test for certain diagnoses. The phlebotomist must know those requirements prior to drawing the blood so that he or she can inform the patient of any financial obligation and, if necessary, have the patient sign an advance beneficiary notice. This function may be taken on by the receptionist, in which case he or she must act on the policies before the blood is drawn.

Radiology personnel also have specific education and licensure requirements, as displayed in **Exhibit 12.2.**[1]

EXHIBIT 12.2 Radiology Staffing

Radiology technician or technologist
> Schooling certificate, associate's or bachelor's degree
> Certification: through American Registry of Radiologic Technologists
> State licensure: through certification
> Advanced certification
>> Mammography certified
>> Sonography certified
>> Computed tomography/magnetic resonance imaging certified

Radiology assistant
> Schooling: usually none
> Registration: none

Source: U.S. Bureau of Labor Statistics. 2007. "Radiologic Technologists and Technicians." www.bls.gov/oco/ocos105.htm. (Accessed 11/8/08.)

As with lab personnel, the experienced and educated staff members are paid commensurate with their training background, and their presence usually allows the X-ray department to run effectively. Radiology has become specialized, and the requirements for certain modalities (e.g., sonography, nuclear medicine, computed tomography) include certifications. Because of this increased specialization, practices often outsource this function to a company that provides the equipment and personnel.

A RN can be an integral part of the radiology team. He or she can help monitor patients, give medications, provide venous access, and inject intravenous medications or dyes. Often, the RN is borrowed from another department if the radiology department does not have a full-time need for one.

OTHER MODALITIES

Rehabilitative staff usually have college degrees. A breakdown of type, education, and certification of each modality that falls in this area is provided in **Exhibit 12.3.**[1]

---

1   U.S. Bureau of Labor Statistics. 2007. Occupational Outlook Handbook. www.bls.gov/oco/. (Accessed 11/8/08 & 2.26.2016.)

EXHIBIT 12.3 Rehabilitative Services

Physical therapy
    Physical therapist
        Schooling: master's or doctoral degree
        Licensure: must be licensed by state
    Physical therapist assistant
        Schooling: associate's degree
        Licensure and registration: some states require both
    Physical therapy aide
        Training: on the job
Occupational therapy
    Occupational therapist
        Schooling: master's or higher degree
    Licensure and certification: state licensure and national certification
        Registration: occupational therapist registered
        Occupational therapist assistant
        Schooling: associate's degree or certificate
        Licensure: most states require licensure
        Certification: must past certification exam
    Occupational therapy aide
        Training: on the job
Speech therapy
    Speech therapist or speech-language therapist
        Schooling: master's degree
        Licensure: most states require licensure
        Certification: national certification

Source: U.S. Bureau of Labor Statistics. 2007. "Occupational Outlook Handbook". www.bls.gov/oco/. (Accessed 11/8/08.)

The use of a physical therapy assistant or an occupational therapy assistant can increase efficiency of the rehabilitative staff in a cost-effective manner. However, these personnel require supervision by a physical therapist or an occupational therapist.

The respiratory therapy and pain management areas of the practice may also have specialized staff. In many different specialties, cosmetic injections are most often handled by the physician.

RETAIL

The right type of staff needed to perform retail duties depends on the retail options offered. Clinics often outsource the pharmacy portion of the operation to a pharmacy company or to an independent pharmacy. Some physicians do provide minimal pharmacy services in their office, but these are limited because many federal and state regulations must be followed.

If the retail product is cosmetic or skin care related, the right type of staff person may be someone who is a good salesperson. An orthotic retail clinic, on the other hand, requires someone proficient in fitting products.

FUNCTIONS IN THE PRACTICE

The main functions of any ancillary service in a medical practice are to provide patient care services, ensure that the patient has convenient options, and provide opportunities for revenue. With today's decreasing reimbursements, the reality is that most family practice clinics have a difficult time depending only on provider services for reimbursement. Specialty physicians are also looking for opportunities to increase revenue. As we look at the changes in reimbursement, ancillary services can be an integral part of the treatment plan to allow patients to better manage their illnesses and remain healthy.

STAFF PRODUCTION AND THE RIGHT AMOUNT OF STAFF

Measures can be used to determine staff production. These include the number of patients, the number of procedures, or the number of products sold. Benchmarking standards can compare your practice to those of like practices. For diagnostic testing, production numbers are easy to benchmark because all venipunctures and tests performed are recorded. Benchmarking with other practices and over time provides a good picture of the production of the department.

EFFICIENCY

A laboratory or radiology department can improve efficiency in a number of ways. Most of the efficiency measures discussed with nursing can also be applied to the allied health services.

PRE-VISIT

The layout of the service area affects productivity. Diagramming movement through the area of all staff may provide insight to improving functioning of staff. Similarly, diagramming patient movement may help improve patient flow. In one practice, opening up the lab area and removing the receptionist desk allowed better movement for staff and patients. The practice found that the receptionist's duties were overlapping with those of the phlebotomist (the receptionist was essentially duplicating the effort of the phlebotomist by asking the same questions of the patients). By eliminating the receptionist and her desk, patient flow improved and moved more quickly.

Scheduling for the service may or may not be needed. For retail, scheduling may be unnecessary, but for nuclear medicine tests, it will likely be required. Lab work or simple X-rays are harder to schedule because these services are dictated by the physician's orders, which are placed randomly. Instead of controlling patient access with scheduling, consider conducting a time study and setting up staffing based on past history. Say, for example, that from 7 a.m. to 9 a.m. the lab sees 60 patients per hour but sees only 20 per hour through the rest of the day. This finding indicates that staffing should be heavier from 7 a.m. to 9 a.m. than throughout the remainder of the day. Perhaps a medical assistant who rooms patients can be brought over to the lab to assist with the 7 a.m. to 9 a.m. rush.

Scheduling parameters should be created if scheduling is used to control patient access and flow. Ask the following questions when determining parameters:

- What should be included in the schedule (e.g., ordering physician, past testing)?

- How often can the procedure be scheduled (e.g., every 10, 15, or 30 minutes)?

- What is needed to schedule the procedure (e.g., past history, past testing)?

- Should the patient bring anything to the appointment, or should any preparatory activities be explained to the patient (e.g., take nothing by mouth after midnight, bowel preparation)?

- What pre-certification is required before performing the procedure? Who determines whether the test will be covered by insurance and obtains the advance beneficiary notice if it is not covered?

- What circumstances necessitate an emergency whereby the patient is scheduled immediately?

In addition, the scheduling parameters can be established by reviewing past scheduling history to determine what worked and what did not.

Chart preparation is somewhat limited for ancillary services and may be as simple as obtaining a patient's chart from the chart area. From the chart, the ancillary service provider can retrieve any results from previous tests before performing a more extensive test or, for therapy, review the chart prior to treatment.

Check-in procedures for ancillary services can mimic those of the physician's visit in that the patient's demographic and/or payment information is secured prior to service provision. How the clinical staff are notified of the patient arrival may be similar as well. Reviewing the check-in process for timeliness may uncover opportunities to increase efficiency. An interface between the practice management or EMR system and the lab or radiology system may eliminate duplicate data entry. A process for late arrivals or no-show patients should also be in place; for example, it is helpful to determine who notifies the physician ordering the test if the patient does not show for that test.

The procedure for rooming and/or preparing the patient for the service depends on the nature of the service. For retail patients, a location away from the reception area may be important to meet patients' need for privacy. For diagnostic testing, considerations include the following: If the physician asks for testing on a patient in an examination room, how does this process work? Is the patient's test performed in the exam room, or is the patient taken to another service area? If the patient is taken from the exam room, how and where is he or she returned upon completion? Communication among all parties should be reviewed to make sure processes are efficient.

Visit

Supplies used during the visit should be organized for ease of use. Stocking the rooms with needed supplies saves time during the visit, and a regular schedule of stocking ensures that few supplies go missing. Establishing a common organizational approach among all supply areas allows any clinical staff member to know where items are kept instead of spending time looking for them during the visit. Patient education materials should also be kept in an organized fashion for ease of use.

Post-Visit

Phone management may not be a critical issue for ancillary staff, but the topic does deserve some consideration in this context. For the pharmacy, who answers the phone, and how is this process managed? For a one-person radiology department, who answers the phone when that person is performing procedures?

During the visit, the physician may order diagnostic tests; physical therapy, occupational therapy, or speech therapy; pharmacy; or optical interventions. The same questions should be asked in the ordering of ancillary services as those asked of nursing, and a procedure should be written so all staff understand:

- Who can give orders (nurses only, unlicensed personnel, physicians only)?

- How are orders transmitted (faxed, verbally, e-mailed, mailed)?

- Are standing orders in place? When can they be used, and who can use them?

- Can a physician's signature stamp be used for certain orders?

- Can nursing staff initiate certain treatments?

- How are the orders documented?

- What items are required with the order (diagnosis, insurance, patient date of birth)?

Follow-up from the visit can take many forms, with the most easily identified being delivery of test results. How and when test results are delivered to the physician can be tracked to increase efficiency. Clarification of what constitutes STAT, ASAP, or routine handling of the results is needed and should include when the use of STAT is not acceptable. One clinic's need to clarify the test result delivery process became obvious when a physician ordered every test on a STAT basis so that she could give the results to the patients while they were still at the clinic instead of having to call them with results. The lab staff were frustrated and overwhelmed with trying to fulfill the STAT lab requests. To alleviate the problem, all the physicians came to agreement on when and how a STAT result could be requested. Follow-up on visits for physical or occupational therapy may include delivery of a report on a regular basis or documentation in the chart. Follow-up on retail or cosmetic areas may be unnecessary.

How to handle product salespeople will need to be clarified for the clinical staff. Using the pharmaceutical representative procedure may help in controlling their access.

SUPERVISION OF STAFF

Depending on the size of the practice, a separate clinical manager may be needed for ancillary services. Considering the many regulations that are required in the laboratory, a designated leader is most likely needed in that area. A physician may take on a leadership role or supplement the role of the leader. A designated clinical lead person can help other departments manage clinical problems as well.

In Chapter 6, delegation was highlighted as a particular issue needing attention for nursing staff. Delegation in non-nursing areas is not as prominent an issue. Assessing one's abilities to perform the functions of any task in the clinical area is always a good measure when dealing with patient care. Competency checks document the employee's ability to perform the functions of that position.

Training of all staff should be ongoing to improve the ability of the person to perform clinical functions. Initial training should include familiarization with all departments within the clinic. Ongoing training should cover specific clinical expertise as well as awareness of other department functions to make ancillary services more effective in performing patient care. Having knowledge of disease processes can also help ancillary services better serve as a team member. Mid-level managers should be provided additional training.

As with nursing staff, other clinical and ancillary staff are interested mainly in taking care of patients. By reducing any unnecessary work or documentation, the manager allows clinical staff to do just that.

CLINICAL SUPPLY RESOURCES

Chapter 8, "Clinical Supply Resources," covers this area for pharmaceutical supplies, medical supplies, forms, equipment, and patient education materials. Managing the supply of equipment for the diagnostic areas takes a higher level of management and maintenance. Required proficiency testing can be a large part of any clinical role.

Retail supplies may require a physician's order, as do medical supplies, and the concept is essentially the same. Having someone in charge of ordering these supplies is important.

DOCUMENTATION

Documentation of the ancillary service visit follows the basic documentation guidelines presented in Chapter 9. The person who provides the patient care should be the person who documents it. Most often, the physician will not be involved in diagnostic testing or other modalities, so the clinician performing the service needs to know how to appropriately document the care provided.

All the suggestions shared in Chapter 5 related to the patient visit can be tailored to the ancillary service provided (e.g., a stamp or preprinted visit sheet or EMR form may be used for a physical therapy visit). Telephone call documentation should be performed if patient instructions are given during the conversation. Procedures performed in the ancillary department should be documented in the medical record, on a flow sheet specifically designed for the procedure, or in free-form. Consents for such procedures should be obtained. Any medications administered should be documented in the patient record.

REGULATIONS

The regulations covered in Chapter 10 pertain to all clinical areas. Other regulations that are specific to certain ancillary departments are included in this section.

The laboratory is regulated by the Clinical Laboratory Improvement Amendments (CLIA) to ensure accuracy and reliability of the test results. The Centers for Medicare & Medicaid Services (CMS) has the primary responsibility for regulating labs, although CLIA extends beyond those billing Medicare and Medicaid to all performing labs. The U.S. Food and Drug Administration and the Centers for Disease Control and Prevention work with CMS to educate and improve the quality of labs.[2,3] Three categories of testing are delineated by CLIA:

1. Moderate-complexity tests

2. High-complexity tests

3. Waived tests

Moderate- and high-complexity testing requirements include minimum qualifications of staff performing and supervising the tests, proficiency testing programs, procedures for monitoring testing equipment, proper test performance and accurate results, and a plan to monitor quality.[2]

Surveying for moderate- and high-complexity testing is required every two years and can be conducted by the federal CLIA program, the state survey agency, or another accrediting agency—COLA, the Joint Commission, or the College of American Pathologists—under contract with CMS. Regardless of which surveying body ascertains the regulations are followed, a significant amount of time is needed to understand and follow these rules.[2]

Waived CLIA testing can be provided in a medical office if certain guidelines are followed. Since there are so many waived tests now, CLIA has offered new guidance on quality control. Some waived tests may include Hgb A1c, glucose monitoring, stool testing for occult blood, influenza testing, urine dipstick testing, or

---

2   Centers for Medicare & Medicaid Services. 2006. "CMS Initiatives to Improve Quality of Laboratory Testing under the CLIA Program." www.cms.hhs.gov/CLIA/downloads/060630. Backgrounder. rlEG.pdf. (Accessed 10/4/08. & 2/26/2016)

3   Centers for Disease Control and Prevention. 1992. "Subpart A—General Provisions." www.cdc.gov/clia/regs/subpart_a.aspx. (Accessed 9/6/08.)

simple hemoglobin/hematocrit finger-stick testing. A certificate is required from CLIA to perform these tests.[4]

Diagnostic departments may also be subject to state hospital or health care facility regulations of the state or those of an accrediting agency, such as the Joint Commission. The state may also have guidelines or regulations regarding clinical lab or radiology testing. Many of these regulations may be found by typing "lab requirements for _____ [a certain state]" into an Internet search engine.

OSHA (Occupational Safety and Health Administration) has one regulation that is specific to radiation exposure and those offices that have x-ray machines. It includes identifying the types of radiation, restricting areas to limit employee exposures, employees must wear personal radiation monitors, rooms and equipment should be labeled and equipped with caution signs (reference below).

Each licensed clinical staff member also must follow the state-regulated guidelines for his or her specialty. For example, physical therapy is a licensed profession, and each state has a licensing board, a practice act, and position statements regarding practice guidelines, similar to the nursing profession. Conducting research to become aware of the pertinent regulations is critical to staying in compliance.

In summary, ancillary departments play an important role in the practice and therefore should be managed efficiently. Attention to staffing and processes in these areas, as in nursing, is needed to attain this goal. [5, 6]

---

4   Certificate of Waiver, CLIA, https://www.cms.gov/regulations-and-guidance/legislation/clia/certificate_of_-waiver_laboratory_project.html (accessed 2.26.2016)

5   CLIA, (for this entire section) https://www.cms.gov/Regulations-and-Guidance/Legislation/CLIA/index.html, (accessed 2.26.2016) OSHA, Medical & Dental Offices, A Guide to compliance with OSHA standards, 2003, www.osha.gov/publications/osha3187/osha3187.html (accessed 2.26.2016)

6   CLIA update 2014, http://ftp.cdc.gov/pub/CLIAC_meeting_presentations/pdf/Addenda/cliac0314/02_Yost_CMC_CLIAupdateMarch1.pdf, accessed February 26, 2016

Chapter 13

Advanced Practice

Midlevel providers can be an integral part of any physician's office. If used efficiently, they can bring revenue into the practice by adding productivity and can improve patient satisfaction by increasing access to care. They can also assist the physician with the patient load and allow him or her to shift the workload. The two distinct categories of midlevel providers are nurse practitioner (NP) and physician assistant (PA).

Midlevel providers can be used in two different ways in a practice:

- Midlevel staff become the primary provider for patients. They are listed as providers for the practice, and patients establish their care with them. Patients may never or only occasionally see the physician.

- Midlevel staff supplement the role of the physician. They see follow-up or routine office visit patients, assist with hospital or nursing home rounds, handle phone triage, and assist with call coverage, freeing the physician from focusing on these duties. In this capacity, they do not have their own patients.

Using either way of practice, midlevel providers are part of the clinical team, caring for a panel of patients along with other physicians and clinical staff.

This chapter explores the differences between NPs and PAs, their impact on the practice, their role in the practice, and a cost analysis for the use of midlevel providers.

Exhibit 13.1　Chart Overview of Nurse Practitioner Scopes of Practice in the United States

	Oversight Requirements				Practice Authorities			Prescriptive Authorities					Joint Board of Nursing/ Board of Medicine Authority
	No MD Involvement Required	MD Supervision Required	MD Collaboration Required	Written Practice Protocol Required	Explicit Authority to Diagnose	Explicit Authority to Order Tests	Explicit Authority to Refer	Authority to Prescribe w/o MD Involvement	Authority to Prescribe w/ MD Collaboration	Written Protocol Required to Prescribe	Authority to Prescribe Controlled Substance	National Certification Required	
Alabama			x	x	x	x	x		x	x		x	x
Alaska	x				x			x			x	x	
Arizona	x				x	x	x	x			x	x	
Arkansas			x		x	x			x	x	x	x	x
California			x	x					x	x	x		x
Colorado					x		x		x	x	x		
Connecticut			x		x		x		x	x	x	x	
Delaware			x		x	x	x		x		x	x	x
District of Columbia	x				x		x	x			x	x	
Florida		x		x	x	x			x	x		x	x
Georgia			x	x	x				x	x	x	x	x
Hawaii					x	x	x		x	x	x	x	x
Idaho	x				x	x	x	x		x	x	x	x
Illinois			x	x	x	x			x	x	x	x	
Indiana			x		x	x	x		x	x	x	x	x
Iowa	x				x	x	x	x		x	x	x	
Kansas					x		x		x	x	x	x	
Kentucky					x	x	x		x	x	x	x	
Louisiana			x	x	x		x		x	x	x	x	
Maine	x				x	x	x	x		x	x	x	
Maryland			x	x	x	x			x		x	x	
Massachusetts			x	x	x				x		x	x	x
Michigan		x	x		x				x		x	x	
Minnesota			x		x		x		x	x	x	x	x

State													
Mississippi			x	x	x		x		x	x	x	x	x
Missouri			x	x	x		x		x	x	x	x	
Montana	x				x			x	x	x		x	
Nebraska			x	x	x	x	x		x	x	x	x	
Nevada		x	x	x	x	x	x		x	x	x	x	
New Hampshire	x				x		x	x	x	x	x	x	
New Jersey				x	x	x	x		x	x	x	x	x
New Mexico	x						x	x	x	x	x	x	
New York			x	x	x		x		x	x	x	x	
North Carolina		x	x	x	x	x	x		x	x	x	x	x
North Dakota				x	x	x	x		x	x	x	x	
Ohio		x	x				x		x	x	x		
Oklahoma	x				x	x	x		x	x	x	x	x
Oregon	x				x	x	x	x		x	x		
Pennsylvania	x	x	x	x	x		x		x	x	x	x	
Rhode Island									x	x	x	x	
South Carolina	x	x	x	x	x		x		x	x	x	x	x
South Dakota		x	x	x	x		x		x	x	x	x	x
Tennessee				x	x		x		x	x	x	x	
Texas	x	x	x	x	x		x		x	x	x	x	
Utah			x	x	x		x		x	x	x	x	
Vermont		x	x	x	x		x		x	x	x	x	x
Virginia	x	x	x	x	x		x		x	x	x	x	
Washington	x				x	x	x	x	x	x	x	x	
West Virginia		x	x	x	x		x		x	x	x	x	
Wisconsin		x			x		x		x	x	x	x	
Wyoming		x	x	x	x		x		x	x	x	x	
TOTAL	11	10	27	21	44	20	33	11	40	34	48	42	17

Source: Referenced with permission, University of California San Francisco Center for the Health Professions, Fall, 2007

PHYSICIANS ASSISTANT VS. NURSE PRACTITIONER

Many people consider the physician assistant to be interchangeable with the nurse practitioner. At times, they are. But NPs and PAs differ greatly with regard to their education, supervision, and certification, and these distinctions are important to understand.

Most often, a PA will have a bachelor's degree. Prior to entering a PA educational program, the candidate is required to have three years of health care experience. The PA educational program is accredited by the Accreditation Review Commission on Education for the Physician Assistant, which includes representatives from the American Medical Association, American Academy of Family Physicians, American College of Surgeons, American College of Physicians, and American Academy of Pediatrics.[1]

Physician assistant education takes two years to complete and includes 536 hours of instruction and 2,000 hours of supervised clinical experience. An examination developed by the National Board of Medical Examiners is then taken, the successful completion of which allows the candidate to use the title physician assistant-certified. Maintaining certification requires taking 100 hours of continuing education every two years and passing a recertification examination every six years. Physician assistants are licensed by the state in which they practice.[1] Physician assistants practice under the license of a licensed allopathic (MD) or osteopathic (DO) physician. They are taught under the medical model with emphasis on clinical medicine, patient assessment, and specialized clinical skills. They can perform any task within their scope of practice and/or the scope of practice of their supervising physician.

Nurse practitioners are licensed registered nurses with a graduate-level degree. Nurse practitioners are allowed to practice as advanced-practice nurses by the state regulatory agency or state board of nursing. They can become certified through a national board of certification.

Programs were developed throughout the United States to enable experienced nurses to practice in advanced care. In the program's early development phase, an experienced nurse with an associate's degree could become a nurse practitioner by taking a short course in NP studies. Now, a master's, post-master's, or doctoral degree is required to become a nurse practitioner. In 2004, 65.5 percent

1   American Academy of Physician Assistants. 2011. "The Role of Physician Assistants in Evaluating and Certifying Health Status." https://www.aapa.org/WorkArea/DownloadAsset.aspx?id=627 (accessed 2.26.2016)

of NPs had completed a master's degree program and an additional 10.5 percent had completed education beyond master's preparation.[2]

Nurse practitioners are trained to work independent of or in collaboration with a physician. Because of the emphasis on autonomous practice and training in the nursing process, NPs are ideally suited to diagnose, treat, and manage disease as well as encourage illness prevention and health maintenance.

State regulation of NPs' scope of practice varies significantly (**Exhibit 13.1**). State-to-state variation also occurs regarding prescriptive authorities and practice authorities (ability to order tests, refer, diagnose, etc.). Be sure to read your state's regulation to determine necessary requirements.

While the length of educational training is similar for PAs and NPs, the content of that education is very different. In addition, as demonstrated above, certification or licensure and physician supervision requirements vary. The PA is not limited by what he or she can do; he or she can do anything that is not restricted by the supervising physician. The NP can perform any function identified in the protocol. Both can provide the same care, albeit from different viewpoints. A brief overview of the differences appears in **Exhibit 13.2**.

ROLES IN PRACTICE

When making a decision about whether midlevel providers will be useful to the practice, it is important to first identify what functions are needed. Some of these include the following:

- Seeing patients—same-day availability, routine follow-up,
- Phone triage,
- Surgery assistance,
- Chronic disease management,
- Education,
- Health assessments,
- Nursing home rounds,
- Hospital visits,

---

2   Primary Care Workforce Shortages: Nurse Practitioner Scope-of-Practice Laws and Payment Policies, NIHCR Research Brief No. 13, February 2013, Tracy Yee, Ellyn R. Boukus, Dori Cross, Divya R. Samuel http://www.nihcr.org/pcp-workforce-nps (accessed 2.26.2016)

- Call responsibilities, and

- Oversight of clinics—prothrombin time testing, chemotherapy.

EXHIBIT 13.2 Differences between Nurse Practitioners and Physician Assistants

	NP	PA
Education	2 years post-bachelor's degree	Bachelor's degree 3 years' experience 536 hours of instruction 2,000 hours of supervised clinical
Certification	National board certification	National Board of Medical Examiners certification
Licensure	State board of nursing	State medical board
How functions	Within state's interpretation of scope of practice, sometimes requiring protocols	Anything physician instructs him or her to do within the physician's scope of practice
Seek independence	Possibly, with physician oversight or collaboration	No
Viewpoint	Nursing model Illness prevention Health maintenance	Medical model Emphasis on clinical medicine, patient assessment, specialized clinical skills

Second, consider what the physicians are looking for and how the midlevel provider will fit into current practice patterns. Will the physician allow the midlevel to see patients? This question may seem silly, but sometimes physicians are not supportive of the midlevel provider.

In the process of determining the need for a midlevel, the following questions should also be asked:

- Who supervises midlevels?

- What activities are the midlevels allowed to perform, and what activities are not allowed?

- How is initial and ongoing training conducted, and by whom?

PROCEDURES AND PROTOCOLS

Once these questions have been considered and answered, appropriate guidelines for midlevel providers can be written. Many states require practices to develop a written document, but even if no requirement is in place, a procedure to define expectations of the role is prudent. The guidelines might start by addressing general questions, such as the following:

- What education, training, or certification is required (e.g., graduate of approved training, certification)?

- How is the supervision hierarchy structured (e.g., each midlevel provider has a supervising physician; however, the midlevel may provide duties under the general direction of any or all physicians in the practice)?

- What differences may exist if more than one midlevel is hired (e.g., each midlevel is individually considered and assigned duties commensurate with experience and comfort level of the supervising physician)?

- Who is responsible in terms of professional liability?

- How often should medical record review be conducted to ensure proper documentation, and by whom? How do you ensure quality of care?

- How are patients assigned to the midlevel providers? Will they have their own panel of patients, or will they see only overflow patients?

- Is there a team structure and how will the teams be divided? by age, specialty, number of patients on the panel, etc.

The next section of the procedure should deal with the delineation of responsibilities by the medical staff, the supervising physician, and the midlevel provider, as outlined in the following list:

1. Medical staff

   - Adopt and review the guidelines.

     Establish procedures for qualification, appointment privileges, reappointment, discipline, curtailment of privileges, and termination.

     Periodically review the policies affecting the midlevel.

     Assume collaborative responsibility for medical care provided to their own patients as seen by the midlevel provider.

2. Supervising physician

     Maintain professional standards by continuously supervising and reviewing the midlevel's work.

     Give ongoing instruction and/or continuing education as needed to improve or maintain skills.

     Complete a written evaluation on a regular basis.

3. Midlevel provider

     Be aware of limitations of the role as it relates to the practice as well as to federal, state, local, and hospital regulations.

     Provide written documentation of work and authenticate as appropriate.

     Inform patients that he or she is not a physician.

     Follow guidelines as established by medical staff and the supervising physician.

The protocols may also include the scope of practice for all midlevel providers in the practice. It is always better to record the scope of practice in writing before the midlevel steps outside the boundaries that the medical staff think they have established. Scope may include the services that the practice wants the midlevel to provide, such as:

- Obtaining health histories;

- Performing physical examinations;

- Ordering, performing, and interpreting laboratory and diagnostic studies;

- Establishing diagnosis;

- Performing procedures, including specific procedures such as lesion removal and laceration repair;

- Developing, implementing, and evaluating plans of care that may include prescriptions of medications or devices, education, and follow-up;

- Referral to outside agencies or facilities as appropriate;

- Surgical assistance;

- Rounding on hospital or nursing home patients; and

- Call coverage.

- Nurse practitioners may want a more generic scope of practice that includes the following services:

- Health promotion and maintenance;

- Disease prevention;

- Assessment, diagnosis, and management of acute and chronic physical and mental health conditions;

- Treatment of emergencies and injuries appropriately as to site of service; and

- Prenatal and postpartum care.

The guidelines may include a standard of care that should be followed by the midlevel provider. The standard of care can be identified and defined by the medical staff and documented as part of the guideline, or sources can be identified that reference accepted treatment protocols. The NP or PA may refer to textbooks they used in their schooling, or they may search for sources relevant to the practice specialty on the Internet.

Another section of the guideline should contain a formulary of those medications, including Schedule II–V drugs, that the midlevel is allowed to prescribe. This list can be specific by medication name, or it can be fairly general by medication classification (e.g., analgesics, anticonvulsants). The medical staff may want to institute a specific refill policy as noted in Chapter 5 that allows the midlevel to order medication refills.

The last section of the guideline should identify the requirements for medical record management. These requirements should address the following questions:

- How and where is documentation done (in the paper or electronic medical record, handwritten, dictation)?

- What are the time frames for medical record completion?

- Is a review of the medical record conducted by the supervising physician? In what time frame?

- If care is provided to the medical staff's or supervising physician's patients, how are the details of the care episode communicated?

In one five-physician family practice, an NP was used to supplement the care provided by the five physicians. The physicians' schedule was filled first, and then overflow patients from the five physicians went to the midlevel provider. Because the NP was seeing patients of all the physicians, it became very important to establish communication up front. Every time he saw a patient, he sent the chart and the dictation to the primary care physician so that she was aware of the visit and the actions he took to care for the patient. At this point in the process, every medical record was reviewed, so a separate review procedure was unnecessary. A certified coder also reviewed the NP's documentation regularly to ensure compliance with coding guidelines.

In another practice, three teams were established with each team having two physicians, one midlevel and three nursing staff with separate responsibilities. The team managed the entire panel of patients—all sick calls and visits were routed to the team. The team was also responsible for managing all preventive and chronic disease measures through visit protocols and population health efforts. Each month, the quality metrics were posted for all practice team members to see comparing each team and their results. This engaged and activated many team members to ensure they worked to the top of their abilities to gain and maintain status within the practice.

After the guideline is written, a signature sheet should be completed for each midlevel. This sheet identifies the supervising physician and documents that the midlevel has reviewed and understands the expectations of the job. If the midlevel is working under more than one physician, all physicians should sign off on this form.

A job description may be used to identify responsibilities for the midlevel provider, but the guideline identifies specific expectations of the role. Make a final check to ensure that the pertinent state statutes and regulations are reflected in the guideline.

REIMBURSEMENT FOR SERVICES

Most insurance companies now recognize nurse practitioners and physician assistants as providers and pay claims for services provided. However, the level of reimbursement for midlevel provider services may not be the same as the level of physician reimbursement.

Medicare reimburses for midlevel provider services regardless of the setting, as long as the visits meet the established Medicare evaluation and management requirements.

With Medicare and other insurance carriers, midlevel providers may be reimbursed at 80% of the lesser of the actual charge or 85% of the fee schedule amount paid to physicians. This reimbursement includes surgery assistance, which is paid at 80% of the lesser of the actual charge or 85% of the amount that would normally be paid to physicians (85% of 16% of Medicare allowable).[3,4]

Incident-to billing is the exception to the above rule. Outpatient services can be provided at payment of 100% of the Medicare physician fee schedule if:

- The physician is physically on site with the midlevel providing care;

- The physician has personally treated and established the diagnosis for patients on their first visit, and the midlevel provides subsequent care; and

- Established patients with new medical problems are personally treated and diagnosed by the physician, and the midlevel provides subsequent care.

If the midlevel provider has his or her own billing number and provides shared visits with physicians in the hospital, he or she can receive payment at 100% as long as the physician has also seen the patient the same day in a "face-to-face" encounter. Billing is done under the physician's number.[4,5] Refer to Exhibit **13.3** for a breakdown of Medicare reimbursement rules for midlevel providers.

Private insurance companies typically follow Medicare's lead on reimbursement. They may only pay 85% of the physician fee schedule for midlevel services and not accept incident-to billing. Check with each carrier to determine reimbursement rules.

---

3   Centers for Medicare & Medicaid Services. 2008. "Advanced Practice Nurse/Physician Assistant Web-based Training." www.cms.hhs.gov/apps/apn2/default.asp. (Accessed 11/22/08 and 2/26.2016)

4   American Academy of Physician Assistants. 2010. "Third-Party Reimbursement for Physician Assistants." https://www.aapa.org/WorkArea/DownloadAss (Accessed 2/26/2016)

EXHIBIT 13.3 Medicare Rules for Midlevel Providers

	Office		Hospital	Nursing Home
Incident to	Yes	No	No	No
Required physician supervision	Direct	Indirect	Indirect	Indirect
Physician signature	Yes	No	No	No
Bill using provider number	Supervising physician	Midlevel	Midlevel	Midlevel
Reimbursement amount	Lower of actual charge or 100% of physician fee schedule	Lower of actual charge or 85% of physican fee schedule	Lower of actual charge or 85% of physican fee schedule	Lower of actual charge or 85% of physican fee schedule

Source: Center for Medicare & Medicaid Services. www.cms.hhs.gov (accessed 11/8/08)

COST AND BENEFITS

Assessing the benefits of midlevel providers only in terms of dollars and cents does not fully represent their value to the practice. They can provide many other benefits to the practice that cannot be measured. One of the most vital contributions a midlevel provider gives to the practice is his or her availability contribution as a member of the team and giving informal education to staff. Another benefit to the practice is the increase in the quality of life the physician experiences because someone is helping him or her with the caseload. In smaller practices, midlevel providers are complementing physician chronic disease care, bringing the patient in for more frequent visits during exacerbation and/or follow-up from hospitalizations. This can be reimbursed at a higher level than an RN.

However, the finance staff and even the physicians need to know the cost to the practice in real dollars of employing midlevel providers. It is a straightforward calculation. If the midlevel provider does not require a separate staff member to assist him or her, then salary and benefits are the only cost to the practice. If another staff member is required, then the cost includes the salary and benefits of the extra help. It may or may not be realistic to include cost for medical records, technology, rent, or other fixed or variable expenses.

The other side of the equation is how much money the midlevel provider can bring into the practice. It is fairly easy to estimate how much reimbursement, on average, will be obtained for a provider visit. Exhibit **13.4** estimates the cost of employing a midlevel provider using averages of 20, 25, or 30 visits per day, resulting in expected total revenue for that provider. Subtract expenses from revenues.

EXHIBIT 13.4 Cost of Midlevel Providers			
	20 Visits per Day	25 Visits per Day	30 Visits per Day
Salary	$70,000	$70,000	$70,000
Benefits	$25,000	$25,000	$25,000
Other (if staffing included)			
Total expenses	$95,000	$95,000	$95,000
Revenue (average $35 per visit x visits/day x 4.5 days/week x 49 weeks)	$154,350	$192,938	$231,525
Profit	$59,350	$97,938	$136,525

Under this scenario, at 20 visits per day, the midlevel provider makes the practice close to $60,000 if the expenses are $70,000 for salary and $25,000 for benefits. If he or she were to have a medical assistant at $30,000 per year with benefits of $10,000 per year, then he or she would generate approximately $20,000 in revenue for the practice.

An incentive bonus can be initiated to enhance the opportunity of the midlevel provider to make more money if he or she is more efficient. However, before instituting such an incentive plan, make sure the volume of business is capable of supporting increased performance.

In summary, midlevel providers can bring added benefits to the practice in the form of revenue or an extra set of hands to accomplish the work. Ensuring the success of the midlevel requires careful planning and physician participation.

About the Author

Sheila Richmeier, MS, RN, FACMPE, has a rich background in health care, with more than 25 years of experience in multiple medical settings both as a clinician and as a practice administrator. She has clinical experience in hospitals as well as home health and physician's office settings. Sheila's medical practice management experience began in the late 1990s when she was a nursing supervisor of an urgent care center in a 55-physician multi-specialty practice. In addition to providing oversight for workers' compensation and risk management, Sheila provided operational assessments to other nursing departments and served as interim manager in oncology. She was later hired as a practice management consultant providing education programs and clinical consulting.

In 2008, she started consulting on the national stage with TransforMED, a wholly owned subsidiary of the American Academy of Family Physicians. She assisted primary care practices to transform to patient centered medical homes (PCMH) and helped design, implement and oversee PCMH transformation projects. In 2010, Sheila started her own company, Remedy HealthCare Consulting, which provides clinical transformation and team care consulting. She has also developed CareTeam eSolutions to assist medical office team members to work at the top of their role.

Sheila is proficient in financial and business office operations and in identifying creative methods in determining clinical staffing needs and efficiencies. Throughout her practice management career, she has managed several primary care clinics and a general surgery practice. Each of these practices has offered challenges in both clinical and business operations. Sheila has excelled in identifying areas in which to increase operational efficiencies.

Sheila completed her master's degree in nursing administration at the University of Kansas School of Medicine and is certified as a medical practice executive by the Medical Group Management Association.

She is also board certified as a community health nurse by the American Nurses' Credentialing Center.

Sheila would love to hear your story. Please email comments and questions to sheila@remedyhc.com.

Index

www.ingramcontent.com/pod-product-compliance
Lightning Source LLC
Chambersburg PA
CBHW081523220326
41598CB00036B/6310